GYNECOLOGICAL ENDOSCOPIC SURGERY

GYNECOLOGICAL ENDOSCOPIC SURGERY

Edited by

C.J.G. Sutton

Consultant Gynaecologist and Minimal Access Surgeon, Chelsea and Westminster Hospital, London, UK and Director of the Minimal Access Therapy Training Unit, Royal Surrey County Hospital, Guildford, UK

CHAPMAN & HALL MEDICAL

London · Weinheim · New York · Tokyo · Melbourne · Madras

**Published by Chapman & Hall, 2–6 Boundary Row, London
SE1 8HN, UK**

Chapman & Hall, 2–6 Boundary Row, London, SE1 8HN, UK

Chapman & Hall GmbH, Pappelallee 3, 69469 Weinheim, Germany

Chapman & Hall USA, 115 Fifth Avenue, New York, NY 10003, USA

Chapman & Hall Japan, ITP-Japan, Kyowa Building, 3F, 2-2-1
Hirakawacho, Chiyoda-ku, Tokyo 102, Japan

Chapman & Hall Australia, 102 Dodds Street, South Melbourne, Victoria
3205, Australia

Chapman & Hall India, R. Seshadri, 32 Second Main Road, CIT East,
Madras 600 035, India

First edition 1997

© 1997 Chapman & Hall

Typeset by Best-set Typesetter Ltd., Hong Kong
Printed in Great Britain at the University Press, Cambridge

ISBN   0 412 58040 3

∞ Printed on acid–free text paper, manufactured
in accordance with ANSI/NISO Z39.48–1992 (Permanence of Paper).

CONTENTS

CONTRIBUTORS

Dr V. Bergamini,
Department of Gynaecology and Obstetrics,
University of Verona School of Medicine,
Ospedale Policlinico B. Roma,
Via delle Menegone,
37134 Verona,
Italy

Dr E.D. Biggerstaff III,
The Advanced Surgery Center at Candler
  Hospital,
5354 Reynolds Street, Suite 518,
Savannah, Georgia 31405,
USA

Dr M. Bouché,
Department of Gynaecology and Obstetrics,
University of Verona School of Medicine,
Ospedale Policlinico B. Roma,
Via delle Menegone,
37134 Verona,
Italy

Mr R.A.F. Crawford,
Gynaecological Oncology Fellow,
Department of Gynaecology,
The Royal Marsden Hospital,
Fulham Road, London SW3 6JJ,
UK

Dr J.F. Daniell,
2222 State Street, Suite A,
Nashville, Tennessee 37203,
USA

Professor Dr F. Diani,
Department of Gynaecology and Obstetrics,
University of Verona School of Medicine,
Ospedale Policlinico B. Roma,
Via delle Menegone,
37134 Verona,
Italy

Dr S. Ewen,
Senior Registrar in Obstetrics and
  Gynaecology,
St Peter's Hospital,
Guildford Road, Chertsey,
Surrey KT16 0PZ,
UK

Mrs S.N. Foster,
The Advanced Surgery Center at Candler
  Hospital,
5354 Reynolds Street, Suite 518,
Savannah, Georgia 31405,
USA

Dr R. Garry,
Director, Minimal Access Gynaecological
  Surgery and Consultant Gynaecologist,
St James's University Hospital,
Beckett Street,
Leeds LS9 7TF,
UK

Professor P.R. Koninckx,
Head, Division of Endoscopic Surgery,
Department of Obstetrics and Gynaecology,

Director, Centre for Surgical Technologies,
Catholic University Leuven,
Herestraat 49, B-3000 Leuven,
Belgium

Mr R. Kurek,
Department of Gynaecology,
University of Heidelberg,
Voßstraße 9, 69115 Heidelberg,
Germany

Professor D. Martin,
Reproductive Surgery PC,
910 Madison, Suite 805,
Memphis, Tennessee 38103,
USA

Dr G. McTavish,
2222 State Street, Suite A,
Nashville, Tennessee 37203,
USA

Professor Dr D. Pecorari,
Department of Gynaecology and Obstetrics,
University of Verona School of Medicine,
Ospedale Policlinico B. Roma,
Via delle Menegone,
37134 Verona,
Italy

Dr G. Phillips,
WEL Foundation,
Maternity Wing, South Cleveland Hospital,
Marton Road,
Middlesbrough TS4 3BW,
UK

Dr J.H. Phipps,
Consultant Gynaecologist and Medical
    Bioengineer,
The George Eliot Centre for Minimal Access
    Gynaecological Surgery Unit,
College Street, Nuneaton,
Warwickshire CV10 7BL,
UK

Dr A. Pooley,
Specialist Registrar in Obstetrics and
    Gynaecology,
Mayday University Hospital,
London Road, Thornton Heath,
Surrey CR7 7YE,
UK

Mr J.H. Shepherd,
Consultant Gynaecological Surgeon and
    Oncologist,
Department of Gynaecology,
St Bartholomew's Hospital,
West Smithfield,
London EC1A 7BE,
UK

Mr C.J.G. Sutton,
Consultant Gynaecologist and Minimal
    Access Surgeon,
Chelsea and Westminster Hospital,
369 Fulham Road,
London SW10 9NH,
UK

and

Director, Minimal Access Therapy
    Training Unit,
Royal Surrey County Hospital,
Egerton Road,
Guildford GU2 5XX,
UK

Dr W. Walker,
Director of Radiology,
Royal Surrey County Hospital,
Egerton Road,
Guildford GU2 5XX,
UK

Professor D. Wallwiener,
Department of Gynaecology,
University of Heidelberg,
Voßstraße 9, 69115 Heidelberg,
Germany

PREFACE

In this small volume on endoscopic surgery, I have tried to bring together some of the well-known experts in this field to highlight some of the recent developments, although with the speed of change accelerating as it is at the moment, some of these may not appear quite so new when the book is published.

Any serious student of the history of medicine will notice that periodically a new invention or idea is introduced which results in spectacular progress in the treatment of certain medical ailments. Endoscopic surgery has been one of these 'great leaps forward' and in the past quarter of a century, thanks to the pioneering efforts of such people as Raoul Palmer and Hans Fragenheim, followed by the inspired surgery of our colleagues in continental Europe and latterly North America, we are now able to do virtually all gynecological operations with the laparoscope or hysteroscope, with the exception of those dealing with advanced cancer. Endoscopic surgery has tended to be 'patient friendly', allowing much more rapid recovery than that associated with conventional surgery, and as such it has attracted considerable attention from the media.

Initially reports in the newspapers and on television were favorable to this revolution in surgical practice, but increasingly we are now being subjected to criticism and any unfavorable outcome associated with endoscopic surgery is widely reported in the media, whereas similar complications associated with conventional surgery go unreported. The popular press and television news reporters justify such publicity on the grounds that they are trying to protect the public, but we know that they are merely demonstrating the old adage that 'bad news sells more newspapers than good news'. Although such hostile publicity may deter surgeons who are not competent or sufficiently well trained to perform laparoscopic and hysteroscopic surgery, nevertheless it can be detrimental and frighten the patients unnecessarily. It also gives ammunition to the many critics that lurk within our own profession, who for one reason or another have not tried to learn the skills required for this new type of surgery. We have therefore reached a stage in the evolution of endoscopic surgery where it is no longer sufficient merely to demonstrate that this procedure can be performed laparoscopically but we must prove, beyond reasonable doubt, that this type of surgery has a positive advantage not only in terms of efficacy but also in terms of safety and reduced morbidity.

It was understandable that in the early days of laser laparoscopic surgery, surgeons were mainly concerned with the safety of the procedure, but when that was established they really should have mounted randomized, prospective, double-blind, controlled studies to prove that there was genuine pain relief and an improved pregnancy rate. The best time to mount such a study is when there is genuine uncertainty as to efficacy in the mind of the investigators. Laser laparoscopic surgery was pioneered by Bruhat and his team from Clermont Ferrand and first reported in 1979 and during the following ten years the journals were replete with report after report of retrospective studies, all of which had vaguely similar success rates, suggesting that it was efficacious when used by skilled surgeons. In our department in Guildford we were as guilty as anyone else and our retrospective study included a five-year longitudinal follow-up on our patients before we realized that we would have to mount a prospective, double-blind, controlled study. By the time we decided to do this, it was increasingly difficult to recruit patients because we had established a reputation nationally for laser laparoscopic surgery in the treatment of endometriosis and, not unreasonably, patients found it difficult to accept the fact that we had to mount a study in which one arm had to submit to expectant treatment alone. Nevertheless we persisted and eventually published the study in the autumn of 1994.

Our surgical colleagues repeated this same mistake with laparoscopic cholecystectomy and by the time any prospective, randomized studies were undertaken the fame of having one's gall bladder removed by the 'keyhole' surgical approach was so well publicized in the media that it was virtually impossible to recruit patients for such a trial. Additionally, even though attempts were made to disguise the length of the scar with plasters it was obvious to the patients themselves which arm of the study they had been allocated to. Surgical controlled prospective studies can be notoriously difficult when there is a clearcut advantage of one technique over another, but in gray areas such as the treatment of endometriosis, where there is such a strong subjective element in the relief of pain, then we do have to use the accepted gold standard that has been established for the validation of drug trials, which is the double-blind, prospective, randomized study comparing the technique against a placebo or a sham operation.

We hope that some of the new ideas presented in this volume will be put to the rigorous tests demanded by modern science in an endeavor to make endoscopic surgery safer and more acceptable.

Christopher J.G. Sutton
Vice-President Elect, European Society of Gynecological Endoscopy

REFERENCES

Bruhat, M.A. *et al.* (1979) Proceedings of the Second International Laser Symposium. Kaplan (Ed) Tel Aviv, Israel.

Sutton, C.J.G. *et al.* (1994) Prospective, randomized, double-blind, controlled trial of laser laparoscopy in the treatment of pelvic pain associated with minimal, mild, and moderate endometriosis. *Fertil Steril*, **62**, 696–700.

STATE OF THE ART EQUIPMENT FOR LAPAROSCOPIC SURGERY

J.F. Daniell and G. McTavish

INTRODUCTION

In the USA as well as around the world, there is now a focus on cost containment in endoscopic surgery (Daniell *et al.*, 1993a; Johns, 1994). Previously, the use of disposable laparoscopic instrumentation had been stimulated by manufacturers and hospitals who could pass on inflated costs to the patients in America (Baggish, 1992). This led to a proliferation of laparoscopic instruments that were designed to be used once and thrown away. This wasted money, resulted in tons of accumulated biomedical material requiring proper disposal and led to confusion as to what was actually safe equipment for laparoscopic surgery. Simultaneously, some endoscopic companies promoted techniques that have not yet been proven to be efficacious for patients and for which the true complication rates are not known (Bassil *et al.*, 1993; Dwyer and Stirrat, 1993). For example, on careful review of the peer review medical literature, one can find no convincing evidence that laser laparoscopy is of greater benefit than laparoscopic surgical techniques available before the dawn of laser surgery (Grimes, 1992; Pitkin, 1992).

Electrosurgical energy has been available for decades and is the standard for laparotomy. Most gynecologists have a justified long-standing fear of and respect for electricity, particularly unipolar techniques (Corson and Bolognese, 1974). Because of this, bipolar cautery systems became available, initially for sterilization and more recently for procedures such as salpingectomy, oophorectomy and laparoscopically assisted vaginal hysterectomy. Interest in America is now turning back toward electricity as thoughtful laparoscopists take the time and effort to understand the physics of electrosurgery in order to apply it to their patients more safely (Voyles and Tucker, 1992). The subject is comprehensively reviewed in Chapter 11.

There are now three ways in which electrosurgery can be used at laparoscopy. In addition to unipolar and bipolar, we now have a new third laparoscopic method of using electricity: the argon beam coagulator (ABC) (Daniell *et al.*, 1993b). The ABC uses inert argon gas to complete the arc to the tissue from a unipolar needle electrode so that a no-touch smokeless technique can be used for electrosurgery.

SAFE USE OF ELECTRICITY AT LAPAROSCOPY

All gynecologists interested in laparoscopy must take the time and effort to improve their knowledge of electrosurgery. One needs to understand the concepts of wave form, wattage, voltage and capacitance, as well as the tissue effects of electrosurgery and the differences between the various modes of delivery. The primary problems with both unipolar and bipolar electrosurgery used laparoscopically is the smoke generated, the difficulty of monitoring or controlling thermal damage and the

Gynecological Endoscopic Surgery. Edited by C.J.G. Sutton. Published in 1997 by Chapman & Hall, London. ISBN 0 412 58040 3.

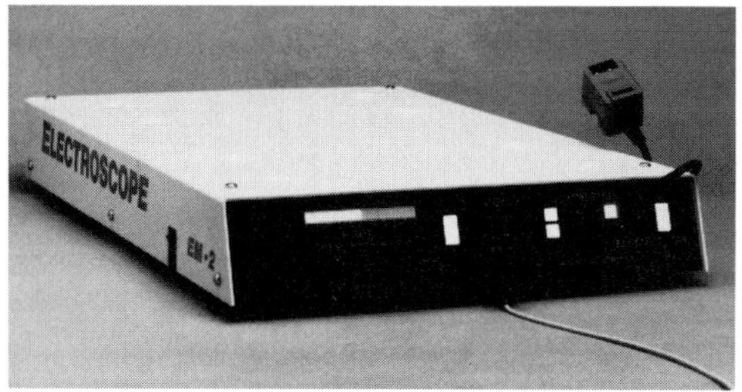

Figure 1.1 Monopolar Electroshield monitor.

unpredictable depth of tissue destruction. In addition, bipolar and unipolar instruments must touch the tissue, so when pulled away, bleeding sometimes reoccurs. With unipolar cautery, there is a well-known risk of inadvertent bowel burn or other electrosurgical complications (Pitkin, 1992; Tucker and Voyles, 1992; Grosskinsky, 1993).

A NEW FAILSAFE WAY TO USE UNIPOLAR ELECTRICITY AT LAPAROSCOPY

It is now possible to eliminate these complications associated with laparoscopic unipolar electrosurgery. A company has recently developed a unique device called the Electroshield (Electroscope, Boulder, Colorado) which can be attached to any electrosurgical generator powering a unipolar electrosurgical laparoscopic probe (Figure 1.1). It senses the passage of current through the probe with an endpoint monitor; that is to say, the amount of electricity entering the probe is constantly monitored, as well as the amount reaching the active tip. If there is any loss of energy along the path from the generator to the patient contact point, the instrument automatically shuts off so that the electrosurgical generator will not fire when the operator activates the controls. This eliminates the possibility of inadvertent electrosurgical burns. Advantages of this system are that it is reusable, sells in the US for approximately $3000 and can be attached to any electrosurgical generator. As

this product becomes available worldwide, it should prevent the occurrence of unipolar electrosurgical burns that could otherwise result from increased laparoscopic use of electrosurgery by general surgeons and gynecologists.

EXPANDED USE OF BIPOLAR ELECTROSURGERY

Another company (Everest Medical, Minneapolis, Minnesota) has recently developed laparoscopic bipolar scissors and needles (Figures 1.2, 1.3). With bipolar scissors, the current passes down one blade of the scissors, through the tissue to the other blade and back up the instrument. This combines the advantages of bipolar cautery with those of cutting with scissors. This product allows physicians to cut vascular structures more effectively and in a safer manner, since there will not be as much lateral thermal damage as with unipolar scissors. The bipolar needle permits fine cutting without lateral tissue heating and without grasping the tissues. This has proven to be an excellent tool for laparoscopic terminal neosalpingostomy.

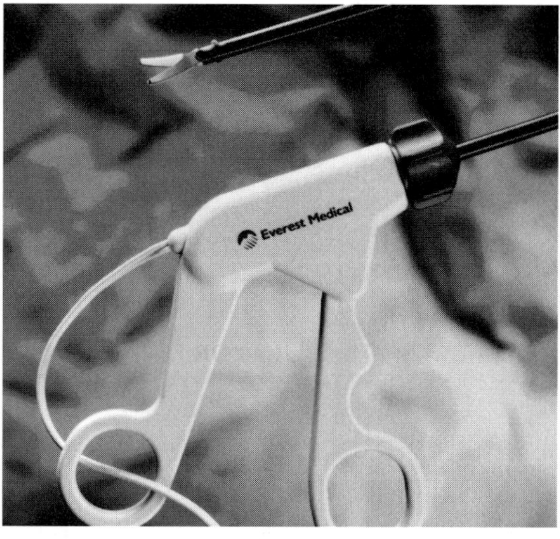

Figure 1.2 Bipolar scissors with ceramic handle.

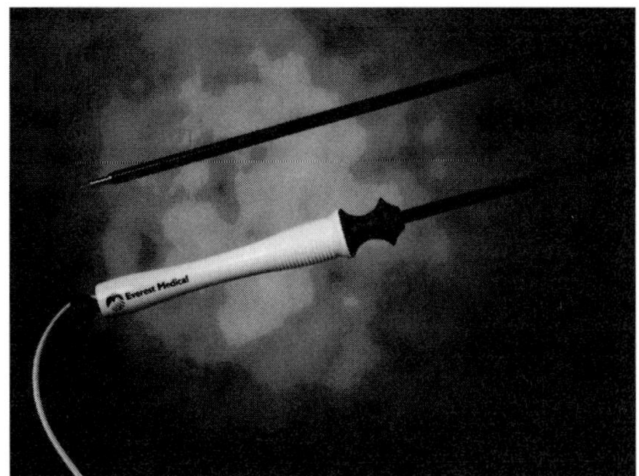

Figure 1.3   Bipolar needle electrode.

There are several types of bipolar forceps used for laparoscopic surgery so the surgeon must use the proper forceps for the proper indication. The type of open bipolar forceps designed for tubal coagulation is not adequate or satisfactory for compressing and coagulating large vessels such as the uterine or ovarian artery. For such vessel coagulation, we use a flat-surfaced paddle forceps that is 4 mm wide (Everest Medical, Minneapolis, Minnesota). As more physicians use bipolar coagulation laparoscopically, they must become familiar with the various bipolar tips, forceps, needle tips and scissors which will allow the safe use of this energy for multiple laparoscopic procedures. All of these bipolar instruments can be used with active irrigation of the pelvis to reduce lateral tissue heating during coagulation. This facilitates pinpoint control of bleeding and potentially reduces overall operative trauma in the pelvis.

ARGON BEAM COAGULATOR USED LAPAROSCOPICALLY

The argon beam coagulator (ABC) is the newest way to use unipolar electricity. This is *not* a laser. Unipolar energy from a recessed needle electrode in a probe is captured by electrons flowing through argon gas past the electrode tip. This argon gas travels through space and contacts the tissue, concluding the unipolar circuit (Figure 1.4). The laparoscopic ABC probe is doubly insulated with a 2 mm space around the internal wire for flow of argon gas (Figure 1.5). Thus, accidental burns cannot occur through the walls of the probe. The ceramic tip of the probe does not retain heat but there is risk from the argon beam coagulator if proper procedures are not followed.

Argon gas flows into the abdomen while the instrument is being fired. Thus, the ABC must always be used with the lowest flow of argon gas, which is 4 liters per minute. We have found the argon beam coagulator probes made by ConMed (Utica, New York) to be very effective for laparoscopy (Figure 1.6). The ABC electrosurgical generator can be set on manual or automatic gas flow control and will generate from 50 to 150 watts of power which can be delivered through either 10 mm or 5 mm laparoscopic probes. During laparoscopic use, the accumulating argon gas must constantly be vented from the peritoneal

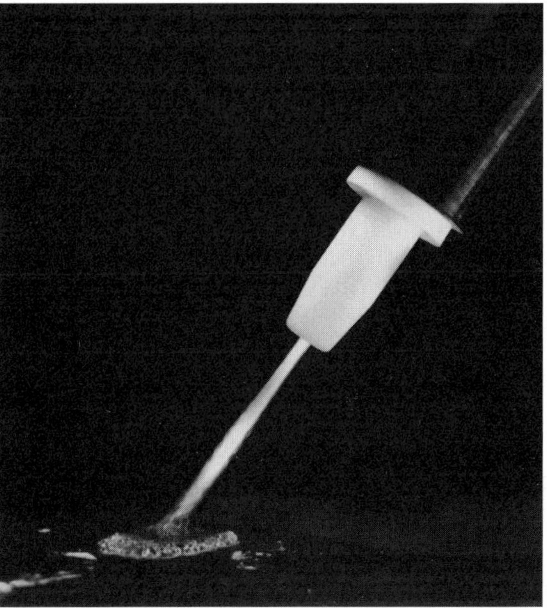

Figure 1.4   10 mm argon beam coagulator (ABC) probe.

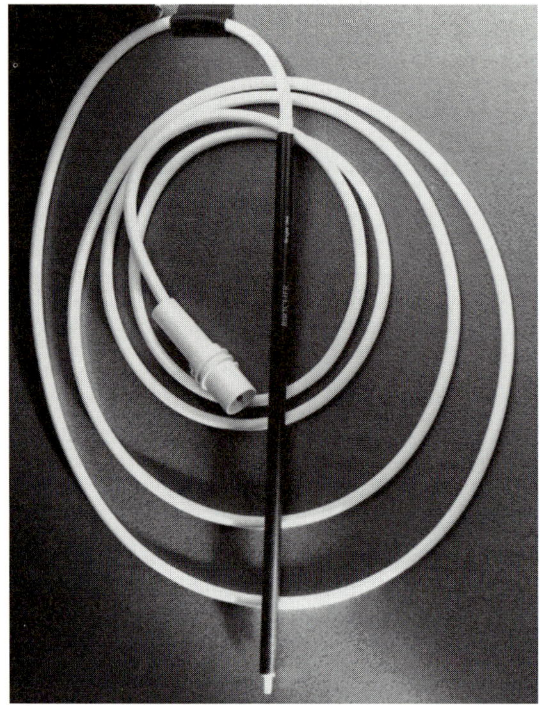

Figure 1.5 10 mm laparoscopic argon beam coagulator (ABC) probe.

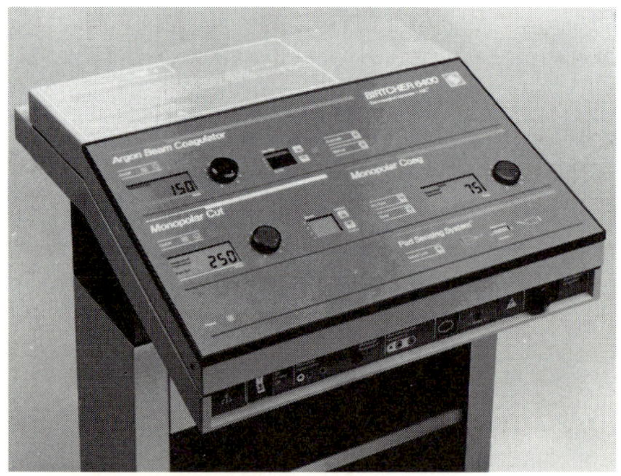

Figure 1.6 Argon beam coagulator generator (ConMed).

cavity. In the past, maintaining pneumoperitoneum has been a problem at laparoscopy due to the need to vent off smoke but with the ABC, one must remember to vent excessive

gas so overdistention does not occur. Thus the anesthetist should always be properly oriented and alerted when the ABC is to be used laparoscopically. In addition, the probe must not touch tissue because of the possibility of argon gas embolism. One death from embolism has already occurred in America during a laparoscopic cholecystectomy because the ABC probe was pushed into the liver bed while firing with high flow of argon gas and without active venting of accumulated intraperitoneal gases (CO_2 and argon).

Laparoscopic benefits of the ABC include: minimal smoke production, reduced cost compared to lasers, rapid coagulation and the ability to see the arcing argon energy when fired. All gynecologists interested in safe, cost-effective surgery that can be delivered efficiently and simply at laparoscopy should investigate the ABC for use in their operating theater. Clinically, we feel that with proper application and safety precautions, bipolar, shielded unipolar and ABC are cost-effective methods for safely performing almost all laparoscopic operations.

HELICA THERMAL COAGULATOR

The Helica thermal coagulator (Helica Instruments, Broxburn, Scotland) (Figure 1.7) produces a similar effect to the argon beam coagulator but employs helium gas. It is a

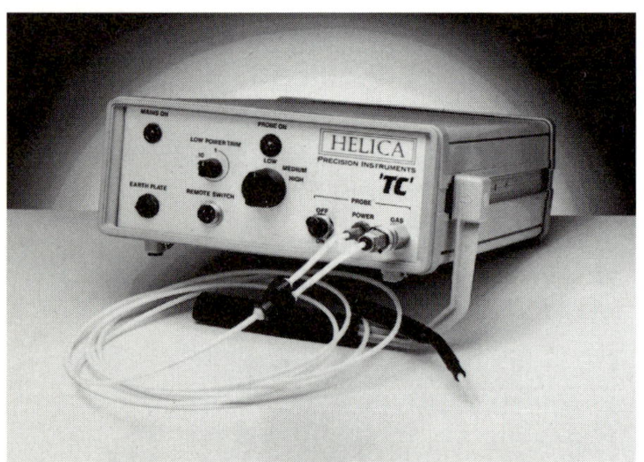

Figure 1.7 The Helica thermocoagulator.

power-controlled device and the voltage is reduced along the length of the flame so only low electrical power is passed to the tissue. The power delivered to the surface can be controlled to a few watts. The depth of penetration is easily controlled by the power setting and the distance of the probe from the tissue, the device is extremely versatile and easy to use and appears to be very safe. It is particularly effective for peritoneal endometriosis because it can cauterize soft tissue to a depth of one cell, allowing the diseased tissue to be removed layer by layer, as with a CO_2 laser at rapid fluence.

When the foot switch is operated a corona-type flame issues from the end of the nozzle with a high electron temperature but low molecular temperature, typically about 20°C, until such time as the flame is brought close to the surface when it is capacitively coupled or directly connected to earth. The corona-type flame then changes to an arc discharge flame which has a higher molecular temperature, typically in the order of 800°C. The flame exists in an atmosphere provided by the flowing helium gas which, being inert, minimizes oxidation occurring at the earth's surface.

OTHER INNOVATIVE NEW PRODUCTS FOR LAPAROSCOPIC SURGERY

In America, there is interest in the development of safe, cost-effective instrumentation. A new forceps system called NuTip has just become available (Marlow Medical, Willoughby, Ohio). This uses permanent reusable handles with tips that can be changed either intra-operatively or between cases. The advantage of this system is that the surgeon can use multiple instruments while only having one or two handles and the tips can be replaced at minimal cost when they are damaged. There are at present six different tips for the NuTip forceps, including atraumatic grasping forceps, pointed dissector, straight and curved scissors, Babcock clamp and a bowel grasper. This type of laparoscopic instrument is ideal

for use in areas where rapid repair of the instrumentation is difficult and the cost of obtaining new instruments is a concern.

Marlow Medical also makes a simple suction irrigation device that does not require a pump or electricity for use. This is called the Pumpvac Plus and consists of tubing with a suction irrigation valve system as well as a vacuum syringe. The pressure of irrigation can be controlled by hand for aquadissection and the suction tubing attaches to the standard theater suction system. This is sold in America as a disposable device, but it theoretically could be cleaned and sterilized for reuse several times. This is a very appealing instrument for aquadissection as it is not complicated to assemble or use.

INNOVATIVE TROCAR DESIGNS

A constant problem associated with laparoscopic surgery when larger trocars are used is abdominal wall bleeding. Marlow Medical has developed 5 mm and 12 mm SAC (Stable Access Cannula) trocars (Figure 1.8) that include a balloon device on the distal tip of the trocar. Once the trocar is inserted under direct vision, the balloon is inflated, the sheath is drawn back and tamponaded against the abdominal wall with an external ring. This allows the trocar to be retained in the abdominal wall without slipping in and out and puts pressure against the abdominal wall during surgery so that hematoma formation is reduced. It will not pull out of the abdomen with instrument passage and stops bothersome abdominal wall intraoperative bleeding by its tamponading effect.

Another new product for improved abdominal wall trocar placement is the Radially Expanding Dilator (RED) (InnerDyne Medical, Sunnyvale, California). This device consists of a 3 mm sharp inner trocar with an expanding outer sheath that radially stretches the abdominal wall to 5–7 mm or 12 mm diameter as indicated for instrument passage. Once the 3 mm RED is placed, an obturator is pushed

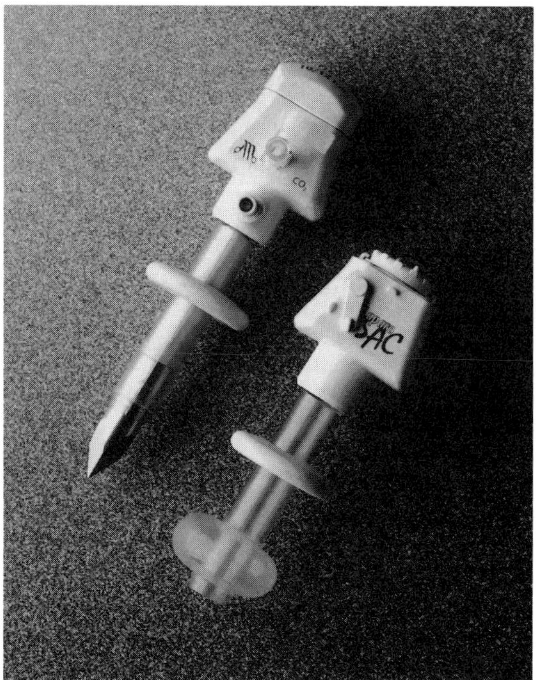

Figure 1.8   LaparoSAC™ trocar 10/12 mm.

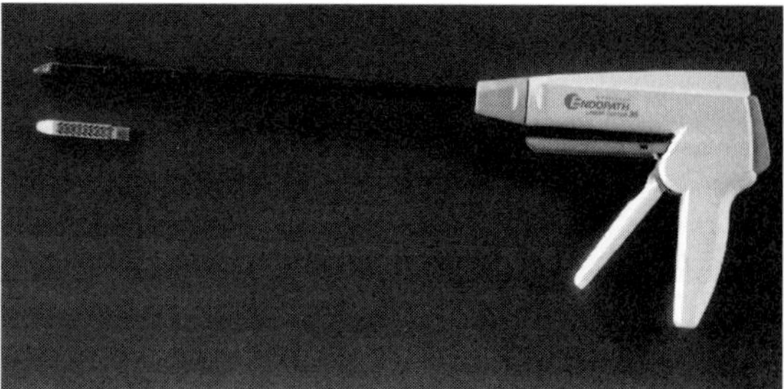

Figure 1.9   Ethicon linear cutter (ELC) 35 mm.

through the sheath which gently stretches the outer sheath to the desired size for instrument passage. These RED trocars with distal balloons are also being used for endoluminal surgery by gastrointestinal laparoscopists who are performing surgery inside the stomach via a laparoscopic approach to suture or excise gastric or duodenal ulcers and to open, drain and debride pancreatic pseudocysts from inside the stomach.

Future modifications of the RED will allow placement of a Verres needle sheath which can then be radially dilated for laparoscopic use without blind trocar introduction. This use of RED technique for trocar placement should reduce abdominal wall bleeding complications and produce better cosmetic scar results with 12 mm incisions.

MECHANICAL DEVICES FOR LAPAROSCOPY

Laparoscopic stapling devices have now become popular worldwide, but unfortunately they are very expensive and require 12 mm trocars. Initially, there was only one source for the stapling device (US Surgical, Norwalk, Connecticut) but then Ethicon Endo-Surgery (Cincinnati, Ohio) also introduced laparoscopic stapling devices (Figure 1.9). To every patient's benefit, this immediately reduced the cost of laparoscopic staplers in North America. Hopefully, as Ethicon Endo-Surgery introduce their many laparoscopic products worldwide, competition will cause prices to fall so that more patients can benefit from the advantages of these stapling devices.

The availability of mechanical devices such as clips and staples has simplified laparoscopic surgery while allowing hemostasis to be accomplished without lasers or electrosurgery in certain situations.

TISSUE REMOVAL TECHNIQUES

Tissue removal through the laparoscope can be difficult. Morcellation of tissue laparoscopically was first described by Semm (1978). Since then, numerous ways of mechanical morcellation have been introduced to aid in this tedious task. Electrical cutting devices (Steiner *et al.*, 1993) equipped with micro engines and sharp rotating cylinders possess extraordinary cutting capability with the advantages of easy sterilization and reusability. Cook OB/GYN (Spencer, Indiana) have developed a tissue morcellator which incorporates the use of a rotary blade and suction system for morcellation and removal of dissected tissue under direct vision in conjunction with a durable LapSac™ made of Gore-Tex to prevent intra-abdominal spillage. Morcellation can be tedious and time consuming and the use of sharp instruments inside the abdomen is dangerous. Because of this, we favor the use of a minilaparotomy or colpotomy to remove large solid masses. Tissue extraction bags can also be helpful for removing clots, blood, ectopic pregnancies, ovarian tissue or other intra-abdominal contents from the abdominal cavity.

If trocar incisions are to be extended to allow tissue removal, we recommend doing this through the umbilicus or in the midline suprapubically to reduce the risk of abdominal wall bleeding. Colpotomy can be done safely by putting a wet sponge in the vagina and cutting transversely close to the posterior cervix under laparoscopic control while pressing the sponge up into the cul-de-sac. Another technique for colpotomy employs a 10–11 mm trocar without the sleeve (Childers and Huang, 1993). Once colpotomy has been performed, the problem is maintaining adequate pneumoperitoneum. Gasless laparoscopy, which allows the abdominal wall to be elevated using a retractor, can allow laparoscopic procedures to be performed while the cul-de-sac is opened to room air. This can be particularly helpful in the later stages of a laparoscopically assisted vaginal hysterectomy. However, the current system for gasless laparoscopy (Laparolift, Origen Medsystems Inc, Menlo Park, California) is cumbersome, expensive and not effective in obese patients.

THE HARMONIC SCALPEL

A totally new method for hemostatic tissue separation has recently become available which uses an ultrasonic fiber to activate a laparoscopic knife blade (Figures 1.10, 1.11). The harmonic scalpel (UltraCision Inc., Smithfield, Rhode Island, USA) uses ultrasonic technology to create a balance between

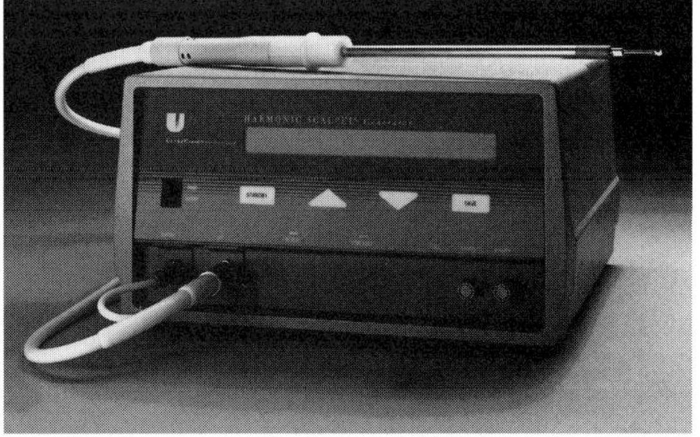

Figure 1.10 Harmonic scalpel generator and handpiece.

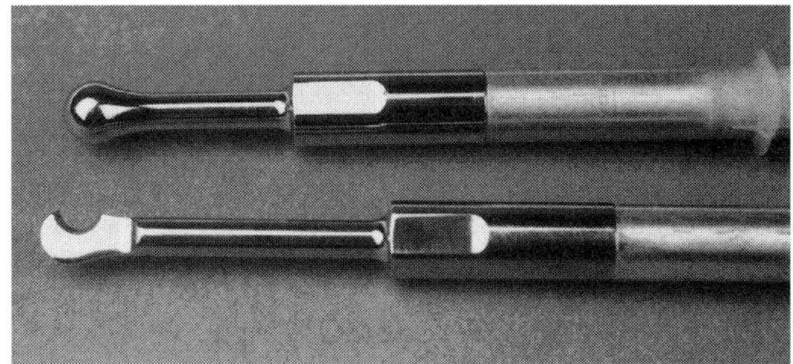

Figure 1.11 Harmonic scalpel ball probe and knife probe.

cutting and coagulation without the hazards of electrical current or stray laser light. The blade moves back and forth 60–80 µm at an imperceptible frequency of 55 000 times per second to produce local friction. Unlike laser surgery and electrosurgery which use heat to cause hemostasis, the harmonic scalpel converts electrical energy to mechanical motion for controlled cool blade cutting, thus eliminating the risk of damage to adjacent tissues. The blade's rapid minor motion causes tissue collagen molecules to vibrate and denature, forming a coagulum that seals off the severed vessels. This occurs simultaneously with the cutting of small vessels. Larger diameter vessels can be coagulated by employing the back or side of the blade to compress the vessel prior to transection. The harmonic scalpel can be used with 5 mm or 10 mm scalpel tips to cut tissue without electricity or smoke.

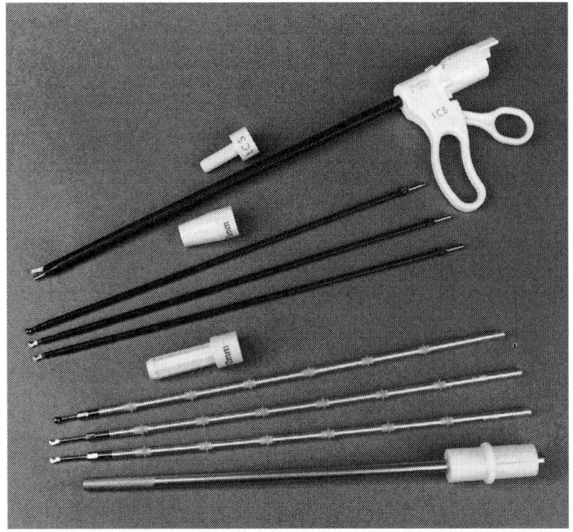

Figure 1.12   Harmonic scalpel and LCS with multiple probe attachments.

The generator sells for approximately $10 000 in America while a flexible ultrasonic catheter is being designed for partial reuse to make the system cost effective for laparoscopic surgery. The company is also designing a 10 mm ultrasonic cutting and grasping forceps which will allow occlusion of larger vessels (LCS) (Figure 1.12). Gynecologic indications cited for its use include adhesiolysis, endometriosis therapy, myomectomy, ovarian cystectomy, laparoscopic hysterectomy and treatment of ectopic pregnancy. Initial reports of laparoscopic use of the harmonic scalpel are promising and animal studies reveal minimal tissue trauma and good wound healing (Tulandi, 1994).

CAVITRON ULTRASONIC SURGICAL ASPIRATOR (CUSA)

The Cavitron ultrasonic surgical aspirator (CUSA; Valleylab, Boulder, Colorado) combines tissue fragmentation, irrigation and tissue aspiration and allows dissection of water-dense tissue away from collagen-rich structures such as blood vessels, ureters and nerves (Baggish, 1992). The CUSA has been used in urology (Addonizio, 1986; Muraki *et al.*, 1993), neurosurgery (Brotchi, 1992; Radnicki, 1991), general surgery (Storch, 1991; Little, 1991), gynecologic oncology (Wu, 1992) and, more recently, gynecologic endoscopic surgery (Vasquez, 1993). With the advantage of more precise removal of undesirable tissue with minimal damage to adjacent structures, the CUSA has been applied to laparoscopic surgery with less risk of damage to vessels, bowel and ureters compared with currently used modalities. Initial enthusiasm (Hurst *et al.*, 1992) was tempered by major disadvantages including cost ($100 000 plus), prolonged operative times and a paucity of data to establish its superiority over existing methods. A new CUSA/CEM with electrocautery function at the handpiece has recently been introduced (Muraki *et al.*, 1993). The advantages of this new device over the original CUSA are more precise resection of tissue, shorter operating times and reduction of blood loss. Despite the development of the second-generation CUSA/CEM and its improvements on its predecessor by the addition of electrocautery, critical assessment of this and any new instrument is essential to establish its superiority over existing methods before making it widely available for laparoscopic surgery.

THOUGHTS ON CREDENTIALING AND SAFETY IN LAPAROSCOPIC SURGERY

Having traveled around the world and presented laparoscopic workshops in varying environments, there is one common fault that I encounter. This is the novice laparoscopist who wants to go on a short introductory course and then immediately attempt the most difficult advanced procedures. Camus said 'One cannot create experience, but must live it'. This is certainly true with laparoscopic surgery. The laparoscopist should begin with the easiest cases and then slowly advance to the more difficult ones, at all times thinking about their patient's welfare and their personal limits regarding equipment, assistance and technical skills. Video equipment is mandatory for advanced operative laparoscopic procedures, as well as the ability to use multiple probes and the availability of good assistance. One cannot over-emphasize how important the team approach can be. A theater assistant who is well trained and knowledgeable and a technician who maintains the equipment and keeps everything properly functioning in the operating room can make difficult operations go well.

We encourage physicians interested in laparoscopic surgery to read the literature, view surgical videos and visit people who are doing advanced laparoscopic procedures to observe them operating. Hands-on training using a pelvic trainer or animal model to practice the technique before undertaking it on patients is mandatory. Each medical society needs to develop firm guidelines and enforce these for the credentialing and training of laparoscopic surgery in all specialties.

In the state of New York, the government has mandated guidelines for laparoscopy training in general surgery because of the high number of errors by general surgeons just beginning laparoscopy. Hopefully, the readers of this chapter will take heed of the comments concerning the need for proper training before attempting difficult procedures. Many well-trained endoscopists throughout the world would be very happy to work with physicians who wish to advance their skills. Many courses for teaching endoscopic surgery are available. However, the best course combines didactic sessions, hands-on animal models and observation of live surgical cases demonstrating the techniques. Most importantly, postgraduate courses are only an introduction to endoscopic surgery and the judicious use of preceptorships and proctorships will allow more refinement of one's surgical abilities.

Throughout the evolution of surgery, instruments have come and gone, being replaced by better, more efficient products. This especially holds true in the rapidly expanding field of laparoscopic surgery which is so de-

pendent upon the equipment that is available. As gynecologists embrace advanced operative laparoscopy, they will not have to experience all the complications and difficulties of the past (See *et al.*, 1993). It is hoped that trained gynecologic laparoscopists can pass on their experiences to others. This should help reduce complication rates, telescope the time taken to progress from beginning laparoscopy to advanced procedures and allow the continued introduction of products that are safe, cost effective, reliable and require minimal maintenance.

CONCLUSION

Laparoscopy, which began initially as a simple diagnostic instrument, has now become a major tool for surgical procedures in many specialties, including urology, thoracic surgery, orthopedic surgery, general surgery and gynecology. The development of new surgical instrumentation and techniques is paramount to the advancement of laparoscopic surgery. Unfortunately, such advances in medical technologies are at the center of the rising costs in health care worldwide.

We are at a fork in the road. We have a wave of new technology and rising expenditure and as a key link in the maintenance of medical excellence, physicians will need to evaluate and prevent the proliferation of new medical devices that have no proven cost effectiveness or improved efficacy over what is currently available. Hopefully, the worldwide community of laparoscopists can work together to expand the availability of safe, minimally invasive surgery in a cost-effective manner to all patients.

REFERENCES

Addonizio, J.C. (1986) Cavitrons in urologic surgery. *Urol Clin North Am*, **13**, 445–54.
Baggish, M.S. (1992) The most expensive hysterectomy (editorial). *J Gynecol Surg*, **8**, 21.
Bassil, S., Nisolle, 4M. and Donnez, J. (1993) Com-

plications of endoscopic surgery in gynecology. *Gynaec Endosc*, **2**, 199.

Brotchi, J. (1992) Surgery of intramedullary spinal cord tumors. *Acta Neurochir* (Wien), **116**, 176–8.

Childers, J. and Huang, D. (1993) Laparoscopic trocar-assisted colpotomy. *Obstet Gynecol*, **81**, 153–5.

Corson, S.L. and Bolognese, R.J. (1974) Electrosurgical hazards in laparoscopy (letter). *JAMA*, **927**, 1261.

Daniell, J.F., McTavish, G., Kurtz, B.R. *et al.* (1993a) Laparoscopically assisted vaginal hysterectomy: the initial Nashville experience. *J Reprod Med*, **38**, 537–42.

Daniell, J.F., Fisher, B. and Alexander, W. (1993b) Laparoscopic evaluation of the argon beam coagulator: initial report. *J Reprod Med*, **38**, 121–5.

Dwyer, N. and Stirrat, G.M. (1993) Randomized trials in gynecological endoscopy (editorial). *Gynaec Endosc*, **2**, 195.

Grimes, D.A. (1992) Frontiers of operative laparoscopy: a review and critique of the evidence. *Am J Obstet Gynecol*, **166**, 1062–71.

Grosskinsky, C.M. (1993) Laparoscopic capacitance: a mystery measured. *Am J Obstet Gynecol*, **169**, 1632–5.

Hurst, B.S., Awoniyi, C.A., Stephens, J.K. *et al.* (1992) Application of the Cavitron Ultrasonic Surgical Aspirator (CUSA) for gynecological laparoscopic surgery using the rabbit as an animal model. *Fertil Steril*, **58**, 444–8.

Johns, D.A. (1994) Laparoscopically assisted vaginal hysterectomy: a cost-effective approach. *Female Patient*, **19**, 46–58.

Little, J.M. (1991) Impact of the CUSA and operative ultrasound on hepatic resection. *HPB Surg*, **3**, 271–7.

Muraki, J., Addonizio, J.C., Lastarria, E. *et al.* (1993) New cavitron system (CUSA/CEM): its application for kidney surgery. *Urology*, **41**, 195–8.

Pitkin, R.M. (1992) Operative laparoscopy: surgical advance or technical gimmick? *Obstet Gynecol*, **79**, 441–2.

Radnicki, S.Z. (1991) Our evaluation of the usefulness of CUSA in poorly accessible brain tumors and intramedullary tumors. *Neurol Neurochia Pol*, **25**, 587–91.

See, W.A., Cooper, C.W. and Fisher, R.J. (1993) Predictors of laparoscopic complications after formal training in laparoscopic surgery. *JAMA*, **270**, 2689–92.

Semm, K. (1978) Tissue-puncher and loop ligation – new aid for surgical therapeutic pelviscopy (laparoscopy) endoscopic intraabdominal surgery. *Endoscopy*, **10**, 119–24.

Steiner, R.A., Wight, E., Tadir, Y. and Haller, U. (1993) Electrical cutting device for laparoscopic removal of tissue from the abdominal cavity. *Obstet Gynecol*, **81**, 471–4.

Storch, B.H. (1991) The impact of CUSA ultrasonic dissection device on major liver resection. *Neth J Surg*, **43**, 99–101.

Tucker, R.D. and Voyles, C.R. (1992) Capacitive coupled stray currents during laparoscopic and endoscopic electrosurgical procedures. *Biomed Instrum Technol*, **26**, 303–11.

Tulandi, T. (1994) Histopathological and adhesion formation after incision using ultrasonic vibrating scalpel and regular scalpel in the rat. *Fertil Steril*, **61**, 548–50.

Vasquez, J. (1993) Laparoscopic ablation of endometriosis using the Cavitational Ultrasonic Surgical Aspirator. *J Am Assoc Gynecol Laparosc*, **1**, 36–42.

Voyles, C.R. and Tucker, R.D. (1992) Education and engineering solutions for potential problems with laparoscopic monopolar electrosurgery. *Am J Surg*, **164**, 57–62.

Wu, A.Y. (1992) Pathologic evaluation of gynecologic specimens obtained with the Cavitron Ultrasonic Surgical Aspirator (CUSA). *Gynecol Oncol*, **44**, 28–32.

LAPAROSCOPIC UTEROCERVICAL SUSPENSION

V. Bergamini, M. Bouché, F. Diani and D. Pecorari

INTRODUCTION

With the recent trend towards delaying menopausal age artificially and the tendency to adopt a conservative policy in premenopausal gynecological surgery, the philosophy of reinforcing or reconstructing weakened or lost functions rather than undertaking destructive surgery is gaining support.

In accordance with this line of thought, we propose conservative surgery in postfertile premenopausal women with uterine prolapse, both for prolapses due to weakening of the suspension apparatus, which is typical in young nulliparous women, and in those secondary to pregnancy.

The surgical technique devised by our group consists of a combined method, performed by laparoscopy, which is easy to do and minimally invasive.

DEFINITIONS AND CLASSIFICATIONS

Genital prolapse implies the descent of the vaginal walls associated with the simultaneous descent of the uterus into the vagina. The clinical classification includes:

- first-grade prolapse – when the neck of the uterus and the vaginal walls remain in the vaginal lumen;
- second-grade prolapse – when the neck of the uterus reaches the vaginal opening but does not come out;
- third-grade prolapse – when the uterine cervix, together with the vaginal walls, protrudes from the vaginal meatus.

Laparoscopic examination in the case of genital prolapse shows the uterine fundus level with the bladder vault and an abnormal uterine mobility; at this stage, the result of successive repositioning can be evaluated by traction on the round ligaments from above or propulsion of the uterine cervix from below.

INDICATIONS

The normal policy within our institute is to consider the conservation of the uterus obligatory in women up to 40 years old and to be evaluated case by case between 40 and 50 years; after 50 years of age, we think that the uterus should be conserved only if the patient expresses a specific desire to do so.

In the case of associated cystorectocele, we propose that uterine suspension should be completed with an anterior and posterior repair.

Cases of urinary stress incontinence associated with prolapse are not necessarily corrected by this type of surgery; moreover, it could cause the occurrence of urinary incontinence. In such cases during the vaginal stage we tend to perform urethral plication according to Kelly.

Gynecological Endoscopic Surgery. Edited by C.J.G. Sutton. Published in 1997 by Chapman & Hall, London.
ISBN 0 412 58040 3.

RECENT AND OBSOLETE CONSERVATIVE SURGICAL METHODS

Prolapse of the uterus in young women or women wishing to retain the uterus represents a problem to which an unequivocal answer has not yet been found and various attitudes are expressed in the medical literature pertaining to the subject.

Apart from colpocleisis, which has some indications for very elderly women without any further sexual activity, the Manchester technique has recently gained consensus, as this type of surgery is indicated for all types of prolapse and particularly for young women with longitudinal hypertrophy of the uterine cervix who wish to maintain reproductive capacity. The operation consists of partial amputation of the cervix followed by a reconstruction of the suspension and support apparatus. It will, however, remove the cervical mucus-producing glands and may result in infertility due to cervical dysmucorrhea.

More recently, interest in conservative surgical approaches towards uterine prolapse has stimulated reseach into new operations both by laparotomy and by laparoscopy. The laparotomy operation which is currently enjoying great success is indirect sacral hysteropexy, involving variously shaped heterologous strips which are anchored on one side to the isthmus and the vagina and on the other side to the sacrum, after bilateral tunneling of the broad ligaments in the avascular area (Minini and Gastaldi, 1991; Farkas *et al.*, 1993; Van Lindert *et al.*, 1993).

Laparoscopic techniques involving uterine suspension by means of shortening the round ligaments or suspending them from the rectal fascia are certainly easy to perform, but are mostly destined to end in failure. Results can improve if heterologous strips are used for the suspension (Harer Benson, 1994; O'Brien and Ibrahim, 1994).

It has recently been proposed, with brilliant results, that Kapandji's (1967) original operation be performed via laparoscopy (Comier

and Madelenat, 1994). In this operation, a Mersilene graft is fixed to the anterior vaginal fornix and to the isthmus after low intervesical-uterine dissection and separation of the bladder. At this point, the lateral arms of the strips are extracted at the anterosuperior iliospinal level, using a subperitoneal tract, the free ends then being fixed bilaterally to the fascia of the external oblique muscle. The operation is then completed with obliteration of the pouch of Douglas and with colposuspension according to Burch, if this proves necessary in cases associated with incontinence.

OPERATING TECHNIQUE

MATERIALS

This technique involves the use of full endoscopic equipment and in particular:

- a 10 mm umbilical trocar for insertion of the laparoscope;
- two 5 mm multiuse trocars with conical points: these trocars are used because they cause less trauma in the separation of the tissues during the extraperitoneal passage of the strip. The use of disposable trocars with safety devices would, in fact, make this passage much more difficult and traumatic for the tissues;
- a curved dissector with a blunt end, for tunneling of the broad ligament;
- curved scissors;
- a needle holder;
- tenaculum forceps;
- a GoreTex strip, about 1.5 cm wide and at least 50 cm long. The decision to use this material is due to the fact that a non-resorbable material is required which resists tension well but at the same time gives very little tissue reaction. GoreTex, with a traction resistance of about $20\,\mathrm{kg/cm^2}$ and high tissue tolerability, seemed to us to be the best prosthetic material for this operation. Unfortunately strips of sufficient length are not on the market at the moment and thus

we advise joining two suburethral slings by means of a non-resorbable filament in order to obtain a strip of the appropriate length.

Non-resorbable suture stitches anchor the strip to the cervix of the uterus and to the abdominal fascia; they are also used for shortening the uterosacral ligaments while resorbable sutures are used for the closure of the circular incision of the vagina.

PREOPERATIVE PREPARATION

Besides normal preoperative preparation (fasting from midnight and enema) an antiseptic treatment in the form of vaginal pessaries is administered three days before the operation in order to decrease the local bacterial concentration.

On the day of the operation, antibiotic therapy is started and continues for five days, even in the absence of high temperature, in order to decrease the risk of infection of the strip. The patient is placed in a gynecological position with legs apart forming an angle of 70° and with a Trendelenburg tilt of 20° during laparoscopy. Very careful disinfection of the vagina and abdominal wall then follows using iodine solution. A Foley bladder catheter is then inserted. After preparation as described above, the strip itself is immersed for a few minutes in the same iodinated solution before being used.

During laparoscopy, the first operator should be positioned to the left of the patient and the second operator to the right; the vaginal team takes up its usual position. It should be noted that the operation is performed by the same team, consisting of three operators who, after inserting the laparoscope, will carry out the vaginal stage, subsequently followed by the laparoscopic stage.

POSITIONING OF THE TROCARS

After safety checks, a pneumoperitoneum is induced followed by the introduction of a 10 mm umbilical trocar for the laparoscope and two 5 mm ancillary trocars at about 2 cm medially from the anterosuperior iliac spines.

VAGINAL STAGE: FIXING THE STRIP TO THE UTERINE CERVIX

After carrying out careful disinfection of the vagina, a circular incision is made in the vaginal vault close to the cervix with separation of the bladder for about 2 cm.

The GoreTex strip is then fixed to the cervix of the uterus using separated non-resorbable stitches (Figure 2.1a), subsequently crossing the free ends of the strip which are marked in order to facilitate their identification and correct positioning when the laparoscopic stage is performed (Figure 2.1b). It is advisable to place a number of stitches at cervical level (about one every cm) to avoid the strip shifting back towards the bladder.

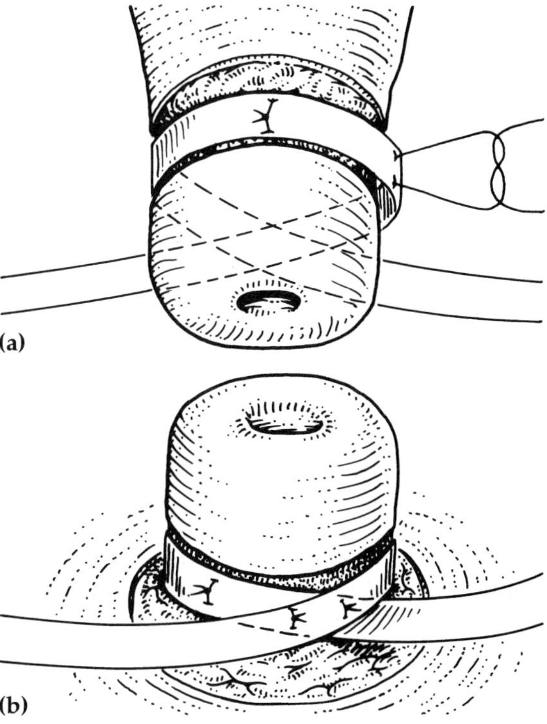

Figure 2.1 (a) (b)   Fixing the strip to the uterine cervix.

The posterior crossing of the strip at the level of the uterosacral ligaments guarantees better anchorage to the cervix and more stability. But above all, if the anchoring stitches give way, it prevents compression of the iliac vessels and the ureters, which could occur if this was not done.

In order to prevent constriction of the cervical tract, which could affect the patient's menstruation, the anchoring of the strip is performed without applying any tension and using a 5 mm uterine dilator inserted into the cervical canal.

INTRAPERITONEAL PASSAGE OF THE STRIP

The opening of the pouch of Douglas via the vagina is carried out using a dissector under laparoscopic control. Then the free ends of the strip are passed into the abdominal cavity (Figure 2.2). At this point the posterior crossing of the strip is lightly attached to the cervix of the uterus with a final non-resorbable stitch. Then the circular incision of the vagina is closed. The closure of the vaginal mucosa must be particularly meticulous to reduce the risk of contamination of the strip.

LAPAROSCOPIC TUNNELING OF THE BROAD LIGAMENT

Using a uterine manipulator, the uterus is moved to the side opposite to where it has been decided to begin the tunneling of the broad ligament. This is to stretch the round ligament. Traction of the fallopian tube is performed using tenaculum forceps, followed by the opening of a small window of about 1 cm in the apex of the broad ligament, between the round ligament and the tube, at about 3–4 cm from the uterus, using single blade scissors with curved points after coagulation of the capillaries visible in the area.

Tunneling of the broad ligament itself is carried out using a curved dissector as far as the perforation of its posterior layer in an avascular area positioned between the

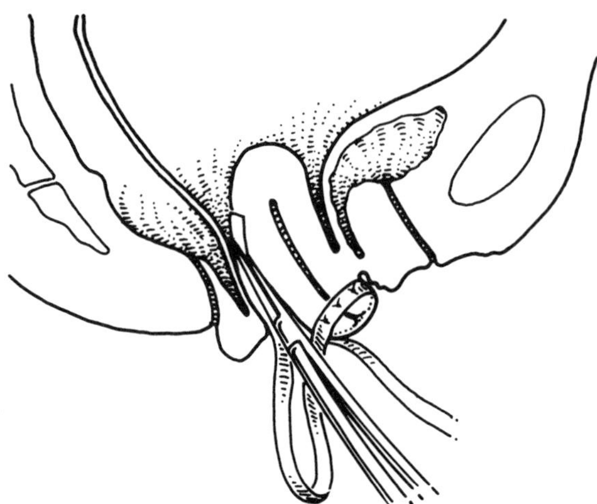

Figure 2.2   Intraperitoneal passage of the strip.

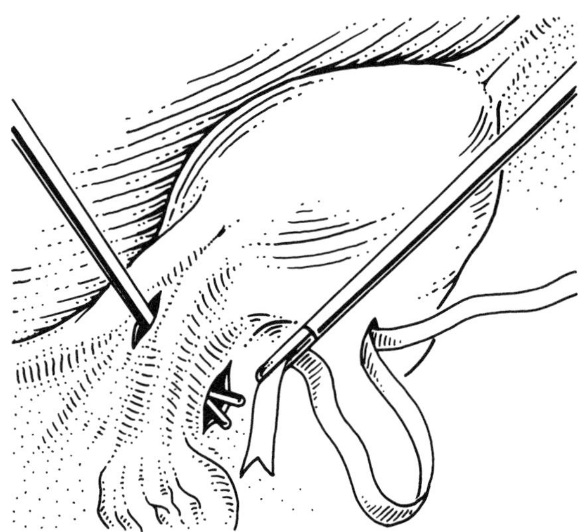

Figure 2.3   Tunneling of the left broad ligament. The strip, coming from the right side, has been cut in the form of a swallow tail, to aid recognition.

uterosacral ligament and the utero-ovarian ligament. The same stages are then repeated contralaterally. The perforation must be as near as possible to the uterosacral ligament (about 2 cm from the end of the uterosacral ligament on the same side) in order to reduce to a minimum the intraperitoneal tract of the strip.

PASSAGE OF THE STRIP THROUGH THE
BROAD LIGAMENT

In order to guarantee the crossing of the strip,
the free end coming from the right side is
passed through the tunnel of the broad ligament on the left using forceps (Figure 2.3). The
surgical stage described is repeated on the
right side using the free end of the strip coming from the left.

EXTRAPERITONEAL POSITIONING
OF THE STRIP

After introducing the conical point mandrin
into one of the lateral trocars, it is then extracted from above the peritoneum, without
leaving the fascia, and is then reinserted
extraperitoneally in the direction of the
window previously created at the apex of
the broad ligament. This maneuver is easier
if the peritoneum is progressively placed
under tension using contralaterally placed
forceps.

After extracting the mandrin, the free end of
the strip on the same side is grasped using
forceps and, extracting the forceps together

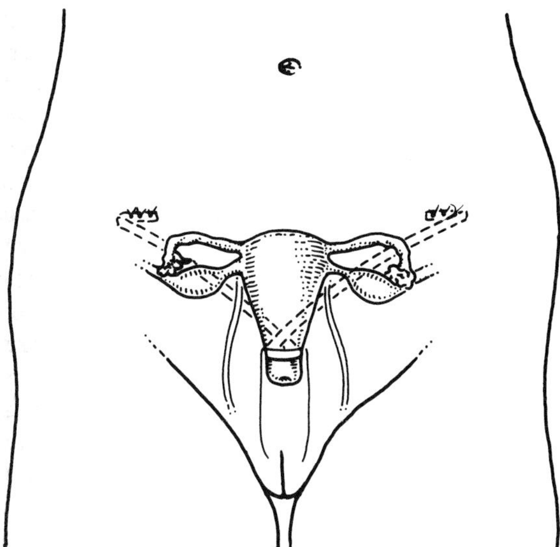

Figure 2.5   Fixing the strip to the abdominal fascia.

with the trocar, the strip is taken through the
skin (Figure 2.4); this stage is then repeated
contralaterally.

FIXING THE STRIP TO THE FASCIA

The pneumoperitoneum is partially emptied
and, after traction tests on the uterus in order
to avoid exerting excessive tension, the free
ends of the strip are then fixed to the anterior
abdominal fascia with four non-resorbable
stitches (Figure 2.5).

COMPLETION

As a complementary stage, we performed
shortening of the uterosacral ligaments and
partial obliteration of the pouch of Douglas
with non-resorbable sutures to reduce the risk
of enterocele. In the same way, even though
it was not considered a fundamental stage,
we performed the reperitonealization of the
uncovered tract of the strip at the level of
the apex of the broad ligament using
resorbable stitches or occasionally metal
staples.

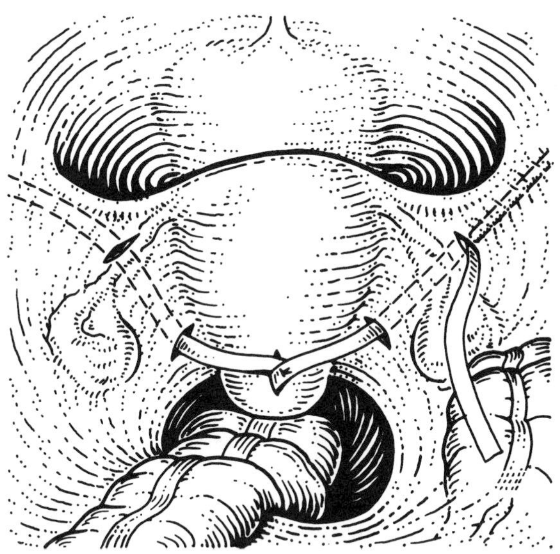

Figure 2.4   Extraperitoneal positioning of the strip.

Table 2.1   Clinical data

No. of patients	Age (min/max)	Uterine prolapse	Cystocele	Urinary stress incontinence & cystocele
9	34–43	IInd degree: 3 IIIrd degree: 6	1 2	1 1

CASE STUDIES

Over a period of 16 months, we treated nine patients whose main characteristics are summarized in Table 2.1. All patients gave their informed consent after careful explanation regarding the innovative features of the operation. All cases were studied preoperatively by means of urodynamic evaluation to be repeated after six and 12 months.

At the end of the operation a radiopaque marker is attached with a stitch at the level of the uterine cervix. On the third day, two X-rays are taken of the patient in an upright position at rest and under pushing effort in order to evaluate objectively the level of the uterine cervix with respect to the bone structures as a point of reference (upper margin of the pubis). The marker is then removed and the procedure is repeated after six and 12 months.

RESULTS AND COMPLICATIONS

This technique proved to be fully satisfactory in the correction of prolapses in all patients as it was able to completely reduce even the most serious prolapses.

In the eight patients who underwent the follow-up visit after six months, we noted slight lowering of the cervix, on average about 0.2 cm with respect to the postoperative level, due in all probability to adaptation of the tissues; the same slight lowering was confirmed under pushing effort (Figure 2.6). However, in the five patients who were checked after one year, this lowering was unaltered, confirming

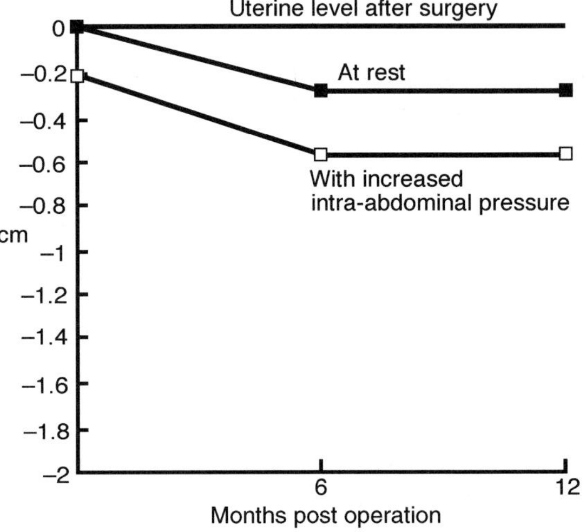

Figure 2.6   Follow-up of operated patients.

the stabilization of the position of the uterus.

One patient with cystocele and another with cystocele associated with urinary stress incontinence at the time of the operation agreed not to treat the cystocele in order that the impact of the operation on the associated pathology could be evaluated. The surgical correction of the uterine prolapse in these two patients did not lead to either the improvement or the aggravation of the pre-existing pathology and the patients were treated after one year for the residual pathology. We therefore consider that cases of cystocele together with uterine prolapse should be treated at the same time.

Despite the fact that there could theoretically be a risk of infection of the strip due to the opening of the vagina, none of the patients had problems of high temperature during convalescence and to date we have not noted signs of rejection. In the same way there were no intraoperative complications due to bleeding when tunneling in the broad ligament, which is the most delicate surgical stage.

The only complication that we noted was as a consequence not of the operation for uterocervical suspension but of the complementary stage of shortening the uterosacral ligaments. This was in one patient who, after one year, suffered partial intestinal occlusion due to incarceration of a loop of the bowel as a result of an adhesion which had formed at the level of the pouch of Douglas under the suture done for the shortening of the uterosacral ligaments. At operation we noted that the intraperitoneal tract of the strip was completely coated by a layer of newly formed peritoneum, which also covered the space between the strip and the posterior uterine wall. Following this complication we are reconsidering the usefulness of the complementary stage which aims to reduce the pouch of Douglas and which is justified in operations where the vaginal axis is modified – which does not occur with our procedure.

CONCLUSIONS AND PERSPECTIVES

In our opinion, the operation that we have proposed presents remarkable advantages as compared to other procedures, both laparoscopic and laparotomic, which have the same aim.

Compared to isthmosacropexy, we certainly recorded lower risk of bleeding, hemorrhaging being exclusively limited to the circular incision of the vaginal vault. Furthermore, by avoiding anchoring of the prosthesis to bone structures, there is no risk of spondylitis or of lesions in the presacral vessels which can be assosciated with sacropexy (Sutton and Addison, 1981). In isthmosacropexy the reperitonealization of the strip is certainly difficult since it implies large tissue separations, while

this is redundant with our methodology (that is extraperitoneal).

From the point of view of pelvic anatomy our operation has the advantage of not altering the vaginal axis angle, as occurs often with other types of operation. The surgical procedures which fix the uterus towards the round ligaments stretch the vagina forward, covering the vesical space very well. But they tend to open the pouch of Douglas, thus favoring the possible formation of enterocele. On the other hand, operations using the sacral bone as point of anchorage expose the pouch of Douglas less. However, this is to the detriment of the anterior vaginal wall and so there is the risk of aggravating the cystocele.

The most physiological traction lines, which do not alter the vaginal axis, are those directed toward the anterior superior iliac spines. In this regard, our procedure is analogous with Kapandji's laparoscopic technique (Comier and Madelenat, 1994), but in our opinion, it is necessary to take into consideration not only the traction lines but also the traction fulcrum, in order to evaluate the pelvic anatomy correctly. In the Kapandji operation, as we mentioned, the fulcrum is placed at the level of the anterior wall of the isthmus, while in our procedure it is placed at the level of the uterosacral ligaments. Thus, despite going in the same direction as the traction vectors of the strip, in Kapandji's technique the anterior vaginal wall is stretched upwards like the isthmus, therefore favoring or accentuating uterine retroversion and making the shortening of the uterosacral ligaments or the obliteration of the pouch of Douglas to prevent enterocele unavoidable. We believe that this latter procedure is not obligatory in our technique, since the posterior fulcrum helps the action of the uterosacral ligaments and at the same time reduces the pouch of Douglas. Furthermore, as it acts on the level of the uterine cervix, our procedure should not even lead to the risk of longitudinal hypertrophy of the cervix itself, as can be seen in ventrofixation operations.

Despite the limited number of cases studied, but encouraged by the excellent results obtained in the short term, we feel able to propose this procedure for that limited number of patients of postfertile, premenopausal age, with primary or secondary prolapse of the uterus, bearing in mind that age limits can be variously established according to population type. If and when this phase is favorably overcome, our technique could also be considered as a potential procedure for hysteropexy in certain selected cases of retroverted uterus. Also, a possible association with pregnancy is still to be evaluated.

The same procedure can also be used to suspend the vaginal vault in cases of secondary prolapse after hysterectomy, anchoring the GoreTex strip to the vault from inside and avoiding the vaginal approach. Our preliminary experience with three cases is very satisfactory. The major advantage is that, during the same procedure, it is also possible to correct large enteroceles, normally associated with prolapse of the vault. In this case, immediately after the suspension of the vault itself, we perform a culdoplasty according to Moskowitz with shortening of the residual uterosacral ligaments, in order to reduce modification of the angle of inclination of the vagina to a minimum.

ACKNOWLEDGEMENTS

Figures 2.1–2.5 and Table 2.1 reproduced with permission from Cittadini, E., Perino, A., Angiolillo, M. and Minelli, L. (eds.) Testo Atlante di Chirurgia Endoscopica e Ginecologica; published by CO. FE. SE., 1995.

REFERENCES

Comier, E. and Madelenat, P. (1994) Hysteropexie selon M. Kapandji: technique per-celioscopique et resultats preliminaires. *Gynecol Obstet Biol Reprod*, **23**, 378–85.

Farkas, A.G., Sheperd, J.H. and Woodhouse, C.R.J. (1993) Hysteropexy for uterine prolapse with associated urinary tract abnormalities. *J Obstet Gynecol*, **13**, 358–60.

Harer Benson, W. (1994) Round ligament synthetic graft colpopexy. *Obstet Gynecol*, **83**, 1064–6.

Kapandji, M. (1967) Cure des prolapsus urogénitaux par la colpoisthmo-cystopexie par bandelette transversale et la duglassorraphie ligamento-péritoneale étagée et croisée. *Ann Chir*, **21**, 321–8.

Minini, G.F. and Gastaldi, A. (1991) Conservative transabdominal surgical treatment of total uterovaginal prolapse: case report. *It J Gynaec Obstet*, **1**, 23–8.

O'Brien, S. and Ibrahim, J. (1994) Failure of laparoscopic uterine suspension to provide a lasting cure for uterovaginal prolapse. *Br J Obstet Gynecol*, **101**, 707–8.

Sutton, J.P. and Addison, W.A. (1981) Life threatening hemorrhage complicating sacral colpopexy. *Am J Obstet Gynecol*, **140**, 836–7.

Van Lindert, C.A.M., Croenedijk, A.G., Scholten, P.C. and Heintz, A.P.M. (1993) Surgical support and suspension of genital prolapse, including preservation of the uterus, using the GoreTex soft tissue patch (a preliminary report). *Eur J Obstet Gynaecol and Rep Biol*, **50**, 133–9.

P.R. Koninckx and D. Martin

INTRODUCTION

At the beginning of this century endometriosis
was morphologically defined as the presence
of endometrial glands and stroma outside
the uterus. Clinically the first descriptions of
endometriosis were chocolate cysts in the
ovaries together with pelvic adhesions (Sampson, 1927, 1940) and pelvic nodularities in
the rectovaginal septum, described as
adenomyosis externa. When endometriosis
was surrounded by fibromuscular tissue, it
was called adenomyosis externa because of
its marked similarity to adenomyosis interna
(Cullen, 1986a,b). These severe forms of
endometriosis have been known for almost a
century as a cause of ovarian cysts, pelvic pain
and infertility.

Endometriosis occurs very frequently in
women of all age groups. This was only realized in the mid-1970s after the generalized introduction of laparoscopy in the management
of infertility and pelvic pain. Black pigmented
lesions within a white sclerotic background
were easily and immediately recognized as
endometriosis and called 'typical' lesions.
Later other lesions such as red vesicles and
flamelike lesions and non-pigmented lesions
such as white vesicles or polypoid lesions
were also recognized as endometriosis (Jansen
and Russel, 1986; Stripling *et al.*, 1988; Martin
et al., 1989) and these were called 'subtle' lesions. Subsequently, with the increased
awareness of endometriosis, the scrutiny at

laparoscopy became more diligent (Martin *et
al.*, 1990) and the reported incidence rose rapidly to over 50%. This led to the concept of
microscopical endometriosis (Murphy *et al.*,
1986) and the speculation that endometriosis
could be present in almost all women with
infertility or pelvic pain.

The severity of endometriosis ranges from a
few little white vesicles to typical black lesions
in white sclerotic areas and the involvement of
larger areas leading to a grossly distorted pelvic anatomy with endometriotic cysts and adhesions. In order to reflect this variability and
the difficulty of surgery and to predict the outcome of surgery, several classification systems
have been proposed. The Acosta classification
relies mainly on cystic ovarian endometriosis
and the revised American Fertility Classification (rAFS) (Andrews *et al.*, 1985) reflects
mainly pelvic adhesions and cystic ovarian
endometriosis. In these classification systems
deep endometriosis, often visible laparoscopically as only small typical lesions, is scored
as mild endometriosis (Koninckx *et al.*, 1991).

Deeply infiltrating endometriosis was recently 'rediscovered'. It is not only a severe
form of endometriosis but, more importantly,
it is far more prevalent than was realized until
recently. In order to review (Koninckx and
Martin, 1994, 1995; Koninckx, 1995) the clinical
significance of deeply infiltrating endometriosis a comprehensive model for the development and progression of endometriosis will

Gynecological Endoscopic Surgery. Edited by C.J.G. Sutton. Published in 1997 by Chapman & Hall, London.
ISBN 0 412 58040 3.

be discussed. Deeply infiltrating endometriosis and cystic ovarian endometriosis will be shown as two independent end-stages of disease. Difficulties in making the diagnosis and the results of treatment will be reviewed.

DEFINITION OF DEEP ENDOMETRIOSIS (>5 MM DEEP)

Rectovaginal endometriosis was described at the beginning of the century and was given the name of adenomyosis externa because of its morphological appearance. This concept should be clearly distinguished from deep endometriosis which was defined as endometriosis infiltrating deeper than 5 mm under the peritoneal surface. This definition of depth originated from the concept that the overall effect of peritoneal fluid on endometriosis was inhibitory and that the behavior of endometriosis changed from a certain depth onwards, since it had escaped from the influence of peritoneal fluid. A depth of 5 mm was chosen for morphological and statistical reasons.

Morphologically 'subtle' lesions, which are very superficial, are generally very active whereas typical lesions, which infiltrate to a depth of a few mm only, often have a burnt-out aspect. When lesions infiltrate deeper, i.e. more than 5–6 mm, they generally have a very active appearance (Cornillie *et al.*, 1990). The frequency distribution of the depth of infiltration clearly shows a biphasic pattern with a nadir around 5–6 mm of depth (Koninckx *et al.*, 1991). This is most prominent in women with pain or infertility and pain. A reanalysis of the database from January 1988 to July 1993 confirmed this biphasic frequency distribution (Koninckx and Martin, 1995) in a large group of women with endometriosis (n = 960). However, some bias in depth estimation cannot be ruled out since 10, 15 and 20 mm seemed to be preferentially scored (Figure 3.1).

Three types (Figure 3.2) have been described (Koninckx and Martin, 1992). Type I is

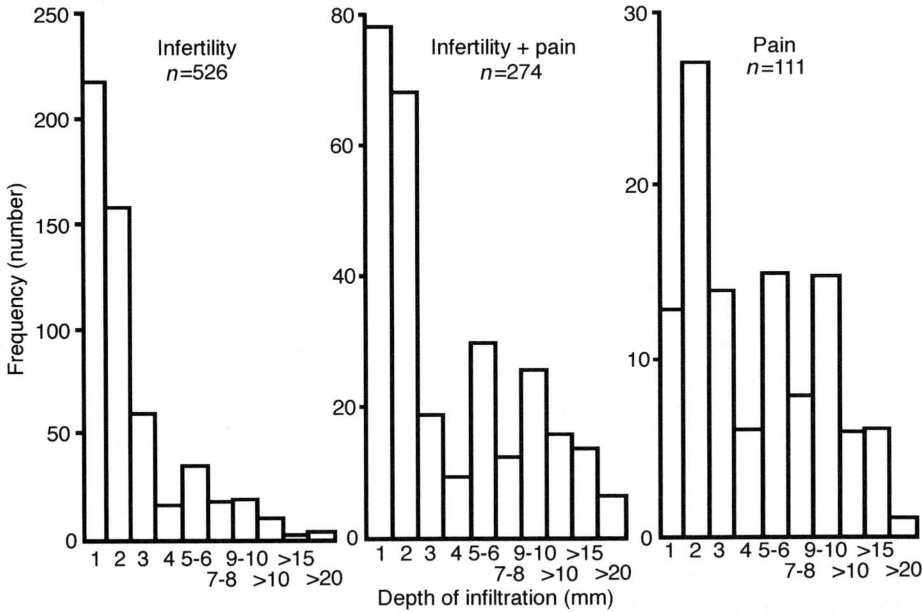

Figure 3.1 Frequency distribution of depth of infiltration of endometriosis in women with infertility and pain and in women with pain. (Reproduced with permission from *Endometriosis – Current Understanding and Management*, R.W. Shaw (ed.); published by Blackwell Science, 1994.)

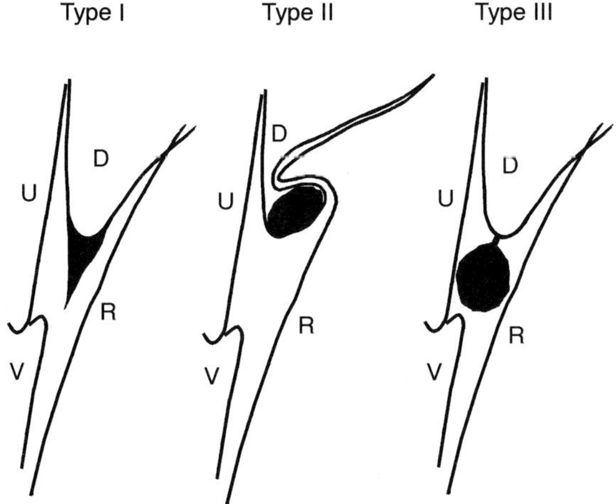

Figure 3.2 Infiltrating endometriosis type I is suggested to be infiltration, type II retraction and type III possibly adenomyosis externa. The uterus (U), pouch of Douglas (D), vagina (V) and rectum (R) are indicated. (From Koninckx, P.R. and Martin, D.C. (1992) Deep endometriosis: a consequence of infiltration or retraction or possibly anenomyosis externa? *Fertil Steril*, **58**, 924–8. Reproduced with permission of the publisher, the American Society for Reproductive Medicine (formerly the American Fertility Society).

characterized by a large pelvic area of typical and sometimes some subtle endometriotic lesions surrounded by white sclerotic tissue. Only during excision does it become obvious that the endometriotic lesions infiltrate deeper than 5 mm. Typically the endometriotic area becomes progressively smaller as it grows deeper; the lesion is thus cone shaped. Type II lesions are characterized by retraction of the bowel. Clinically they are recognized by the obvious bowel retraction around a small typical lesion. In some women, however, no endometriosis can be seen through the laparoscope and the bowel retraction is the only clinical sign. Diagnosis is generally not too difficult since during laparoscopy the retraction, under which an induration is felt, is obvious. In some women, however, the retraction is minimal and the induration can be hardly felt. Only during excision does the endometriotic nodule become apparent, emphasizing the need for a preoperative diag-

nosis and training in recognizing these lesions. Type III lesions are spherical, endometriotic, painful nodules in the rectovaginal septum. At laparoscopy they generally present as a small typical lesion and in some women a careful vaginal examination reveals some dark blue cysts (3–4 mm) in the fornix posterior. Type III lesions are the most severe and they often spread laterally up and around the uterine artery, sometimes causing sclerosis around the ureter. The spread along the uterine artery can be so obvious that this can be considered as an indirect argument for the hypothesis that deep endometriosis has escaped from the inhibitory influence of peritoneal fluid and is mainly under peripheral circulation control. While being prominent in most women, these lesions are very often missed, as will be discussed later.

A NEW MODEL DESCRIBING THE PROGRESSION OF ENDOMETRIOSIS TO ENDOMETRIOTIC DISEASE (FIGURE 3.3)

SUBTLE, NON-PIGMENTED LESIONS AND REMODELING OF ENDOMETRIOSIS

Retrograde menstruation has been recognized as an almost universal phenomenon. Endometrial cells were found in peritoneal fluid in more than 70% of women, whether they had endometriosis or not (Koninckx *et al.*, 1980a), and the incidence decreased progressively towards the end of the menstrual cycle. This observation has been confirmed and extended by several authors showing that these endometrial cells found in the peritoneal cavity were viable and could be grown *in vitro* (Badawy *et al.*, 1984; Bartosik *et al.*, 1986; Kruitwagen *et al.*, 1991). In 1977 at the FIGO conference in Tokyo (Koninckx and Brosens, 1977), delegates were already starting to question why these cells do not implant in all women and thus why all women do not develop endometriosis. The preferential localization of endometriosis in the pouch of Douglas was considered consistent with the implantation theory because of gravity. The

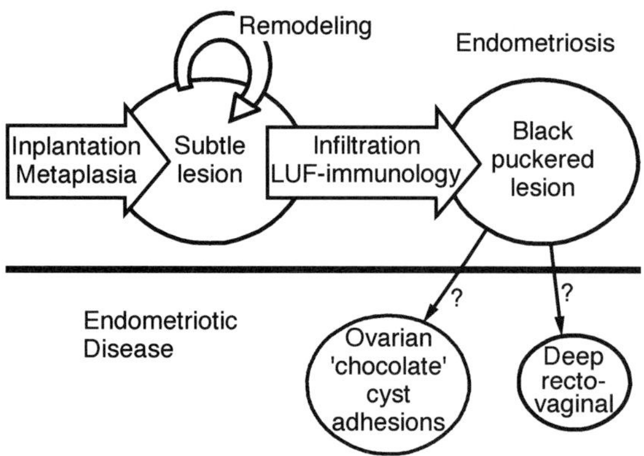

Figure 3.3   A model for endometriosis. This emphasizes the presence of subtle endometriosis in (almost) all women and active remodeling. Superficial infiltration to burnt-out typical lesions, which are morphologically inactive, is quite frequent. In some women endometriosis develops into endometriotic disease with severe lesions, either cystic ovarian endometriosis or deep endometriosis or both. (Reproduced by permission of Oxford University Press from *Human Reprod* 1994, **9**, 2202–11.)

localization around the fimbrial ends has been considered by some as an argument in favor of metaplasia (Jenkins *et al.*, 1986). Both mechanisms, implantation of regurgitated cells and metaplastic induction of endometriosis by menstrual debris, have been proved experimentally (El Mahgoub and Yaseen, 1980; D'Hooge *et al.*, 1995).

It seems logical that non-pigmented and subtle lesions, such as white or red vesicles, polypoid and flamelike lesions, are the early stages of endometriosis because of their macroscopical appearance, the absence of extensive surrounding sclerosis and the fact that they are morphologically very active. Moreover, the observation that their incidence decreases with age (Redwine, 1987; Koninckx *et al.*, 1991) lends further support to the concept that subtle lesions constitute early stages. In order to understand why endometriosis develops in some women, implantation or metaplasia were considered as the key factors and several mechanisms controlling the implantation of endometrial cells and/or the induction of metaplasia have been proposed. Firstly, since endometriosis is almost universally found in women with cervical occlusion and since endometriosis can be induced in baboons by cervical occlusion (D'Hooge *et al.*, 1994), the amount of retrograde menstruation was suggested to be more important. Since women with endometriosis have a less competent uterotubal sphincter mechanism as evaluated by uterotubal pressure profiles (Ayers and Friedenstab, 1985) and by uterine flushings (Bartosik *et al.*, 1986; Kruitwagen *et al.*, 1991), this mechanism could be important. Secondly, it has been postulated that the luteinized unruptured follicle syndrome could facilitate the development of endometriosis (Koninckx *et al.*, 1980a) since in these women the peritoneal fluid concentrations of 17β-estradiol and of progesterone were much lower following ovulation (Koninckx *et al.*, 1980b,c). The underlying assumption was that high progesterone concentrations would be deleterious for the implantation/survival/proliferation of regurgitated endometrial cells. Thirdly, if the peritoneal fluid is considered as a garbage collection and disposal system, endometriosis would become a consequence of insufficient disposal by macrophages (Evers, 1993) or of decreased natural killer cell activity (Oosterlynck *et al.*, 1992). Finally, since in women with endometriosis peritoneal fluid contains more activated macrophages, which secrete a range of products such as growth factors and cytokines, these concentrations have been suggested as controlling mechanisms (Haney *et al.*, 1981; Badawy *et al.*, 1984; Olive *et al.*, 1985; Fakih *et al.*, 1987; Halme *et al.*, 1987; Syrop and Halme, 1987; Eisermann *et al.*, 1988; Halme, 1989; Weinberg *et al.*, 1991; Haney, 1993; Oosterlynck *et al.*, 1993).

Until recently, endometriosis was considered static and/or slowly progressive. Once the bridge of implantation was crossed, these endometrial cells would progress to more severe forms of endometriosis. Only recently has the important remodeling of endometriosis been recognized. In young fertile baboons, spontaneous endometriosis – almost all subtle lesions – was found in 23% (D'Hooge *et al.*, 1991). At subsequent laparoscopy some of the initial lesions had disappeared but new lesions had formed (D'Hooge *et al.*, 1992). More important, however, was the observation that some animals with endometriosis had become normal, whereas others which had been normal at the first laparoscopy had developed endometriosis. Also, an active remodeling between typical powder black lesions and subtle lesions was documented. Spontaneous resolution of typical lesions, however, has not been observed. A similar remodeling in women has been suggested (Hoshiai *et al.*, 1993; Wiegerinck *et al.*, 1993), reinforcing the idea that subtle endometriosis should not be considered as a stable but as a very dynamic situation.

IS MINIMAL ENDOMETRIOSIS A NORMAL CONDITION OCCURRING INTERMITTENTLY IN ALL WOMEN? (VERCELLINI *ET AL.*, 1992; KONINCKX, 1994A,B; KONINCKX *ET AL.*, 1994)

The concept of active remodeling of subtle lesions was reinforced during successive laparoscopies in the baboon, showing that not only can endometriotic lesions disappear and reappear spontaneously, but also that animals with endometriosis can become normal and vice versa, thus suggesting that subtle endometriosis can occur intermittently in all higher primates.

It is important to realize that there is no contradiction between this concept and the reported incidences of endometriosis in women, which vary between 5% and 20% in normal women (Shaw, 1992) and up to more than 60% in women with infertility and/or pelvic pain (Koninckx *et al.*, 1991). These incidences describe the percentage of women having lesions at any one moment. If endometriosis is considered as a dynamic process, these numbers can be interpreted as the percentage of time that each individual woman

has lesions. The importance of this concept lies in the fact that subtle endometriosis could be regarded as a 'normal' condition occurring intermittently in all women. The question 'Why do endometrial cells implant in some women only?' would thus change to 'Why do subtle lesions disappear spontaneously in some women and progress to more severe stages in other women?'. This also questions the rationale of treatment of subtle lesions (Evers, 1989) except to prevent progression.

PROGRESSION OF ENDOMETRIOSIS TO ENDOMETRIOTIC DISEASE

Progression of subtle lesions to typical lesions and ultimately to severe endometriosis, deep lesions or cystic ovarian endometriosis seems logical and is now widely accepted. The evidence to support this is rather scarce, however. In the baboon an overall progression was demonstrated during consecutive laparoscopies (D'Hooge *et al.*, 1992). In the human Thomas and Cooke (1987) found a slight increase in typical lesions over a six-month period and recently Hoshiai *et al.* (1993) demonstrated progression of disease in four out of seven women whereas in three the lesions remained unchanged or had decreased. Another argument in favor of progression of disease can be derived from the observation that the incidence of subtle lesions decreases with age (Redwine, 1987; Koninckx *et al.*, 1991), whereas the incidence of typical lesions, deep lesions and cystic ovarian endometriosis increases with age (Koninckx *et al.*, 1991) (Figure 3.4). The relative incidences of lesions suggest that in many women superficial lesions start to infiltrate, but that this is generally controlled by the defense mechanisms of the body. These lesions will show as morphologically inactive, typical, black puckered lesions surrounded by sclerosis. In a minority of women, some 20–30% (Koninckx *et al.*, 1991), deeper infiltration occurs or cystic ovarian endometriosis develops.

Whereas it has been speculated that growth

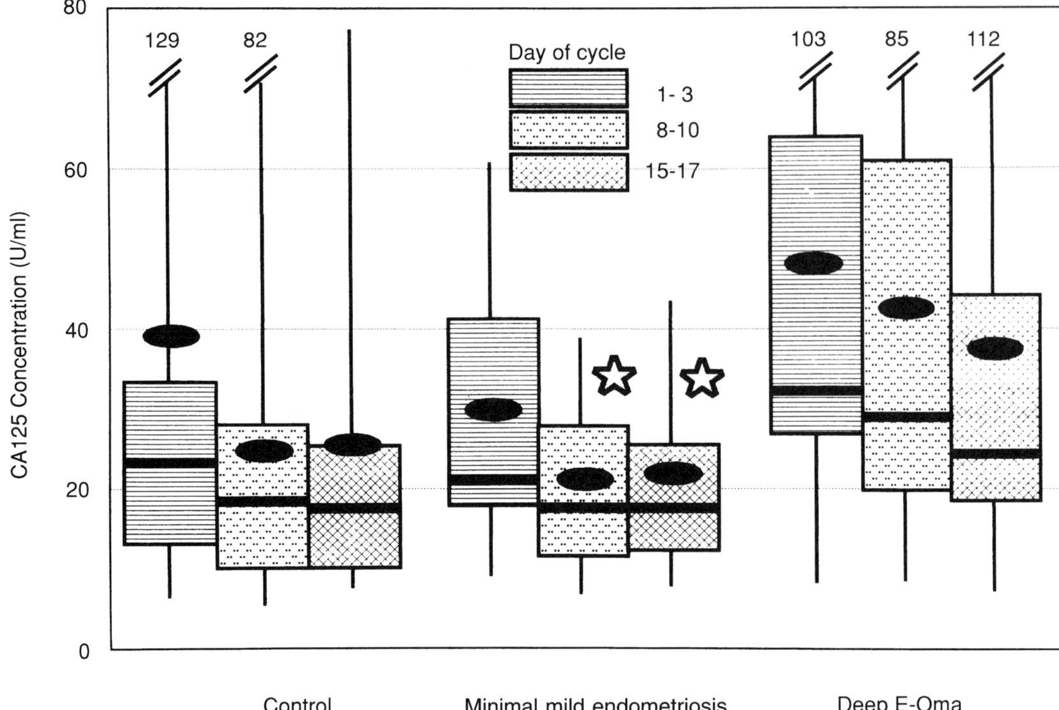

Figure 3.4 Plasma CA125 concentrations during menstruation (▨), during the mid-follicular phase (▨) and the early luteal phase (▨) in women without endometriosis, with minimal or mild endometriosis and with deeply infiltrating endometriosis or cystic ovarian endometriosis (E-oma). Box plots depicting the mean (●), median (■) and the 25–75th and the 10–90th percentiles are shown; if the 90th percentile is outside the scale, the individual values are given. (*p < 0.05 versus concentrations on day 1–3.)

factors and other macrophage secretion products in peritoneal fluid could promote the growth of endometriosis, the observation that the extent of endometriotic implants correlates *inversely* with markers of peritoneal inflammation suggests that peritoneal fluid actually has an inhibiting instead of a stimulating effect upon the development and growth of endometriosis (Haney and Weinberg, 1988). This has led to the hypothesis that superficial endometriotic implants are mainly under inhibitory peritoneal fluid control, whereas deeper lesions have escaped from the influence of peritoneal fluid (Koninckx and Martin, 1994, 1995). Hence they become more active and start growing deeper. This can explain the biphasic frequency distribution (Koninckx *et al.*, 1991) with a transition zone – i.e. where the influence of peritoneal fluid shifts to the peripheral circulation – around 5–6 mm. This hypothesis is consistent with the observation that superficial lesions secrete CA125 and PP14 mainly towards the peritoneal cavity whereas deep lesions secrete these substances mainly towards the bloodstream (Koninckx *et al.*, 1992). This concept could explain the decreased cellular immunity (Dmowski *et al.*, 1981) and natural killer cell activity in the plasma of women with cystic ovarian endometriosis or deep endometriosis (Oosterlynck *et al.*, 1991) whereas in women with minimal endometriosis the cellular immunity is comparable with women without endometriosis. Finally, it is important to note that cystic ovarian endometriosis has also escaped from peritoneal fluid control.

In order to contrast subtle endometriosis, which can be considered as a natural condition which occurs intermittently in most, if not all, women, with the more severe forms of endometriosis which are definitively a disease entity, the term 'endometriotic disease' has been proposed to designate deep endometriosis and cystic ovarian endometriosis (Koninckx, 1994a,b; Koninckx *et al.*, 1994).

DEEP ENDOMETRIOSIS AND CYSTIC OVARIAN ENDOMETRIOSIS ARE TWO DISTINCT PATHOLOGIES

Both deep endometriosis and cystic ovarian endometriosis are end-stages of endometriosis. Several arguments suggest, however, that they are two distinct variants of the same disease. Both deep infiltrating endometriosis and cystic ovarian endometriosis are two independent variables predicting the increased plasma concentrations of CA125 and of PP14 (Koninckx *et al.*, 1992), decreased plasma NK cell activity (Oosterlynck *et al.*, 1991), pelvic pain (Koninckx *et al.*, 1991) and subsequent fertility. Cystic ovarian endometriosis is strongly associated with pelvic adhesions whereas deep infiltrating endometriosis is not. Since adhesions are heavily scored in the revised American Fertility Classification, this explains why women with cystic ovarian endometriosis are almost invariably in rAFS classes III and IV, whereas deep infiltrating endometriosis is most frequently found in rAFS classes I and II (Koninckx *et al.*, 1991).

If deep infiltrating endometriosis and cystic ovarian endometriosis are two distinct entities, the model for the progression of endometriosis should be understood as follows. Instead of progressing to 'severe disease', endometriosis progresses in some women to cystic ovarian disease and pelvic adhesions and in other women to deeply infiltrating disease and sometimes to both stages of severe disease in the same women. It remains unknown which mechanisms control the development of endometriosis in one or both directions.

CLINICAL APPEARANCE AND DIAGNOSIS

Deep endometriosis is almost exclusively localized in the pouch of Douglas and/or the uterosacral ligaments and occasionally in the uterovesical fold (Martin *et al.*, 1989; Koninckx *et al.*, 1991; Donnez *et al.*, 1995).

The diagnosis of deep endometriosis can be obvious at clinical examination, at vaginal inspection or during laparoscopic excision. During vaginal examination deep endometriosis can be felt as generally painful indurations in the uterosacral ligaments or in the pouch of Douglas. It requires careful vaginal inspection to diagnose the dark blue cysts in the posterior fornix because during a routine examination these lesions are easily overlooked, being hidden under the posterior blade of the speculum. In some women the cervix has to be pulled anteriorly before they become visible. In our experience, many vaginal lesions have been diagnosed only when, during endoscopic excision, it is necessary to excise part of the vaginal wall. During laparoscopy type I lesions are readily recognized as endometriosis but the depth of the infiltration becomes apparent only during excision, emphasizing the need for careful excisional techniques when removing larger areas of endometriosis, especially those overlying zones of induration. In some women with type II or III lesions even a careful laparoscopic inspection does not reveal any endometriosis and the only guidance is the induration felt by clinical examination and/or during laparoscopic palpation.

The most powerful diagnostic tool was recently shown to be a clinical examination during menstruation (Ripps and Martin, 1991; Koninckx *et al.*, 1996). A routine clinical examination during the menstrual cycle was a poor predictor of deep endometriosis since in a retrospective analysis more than half of the lesions had been missed. Even lesions infiltrating for more than 15 mm or larger than 3 cm^2 were missed in some 40% of women. If in some women with deep endometriosis type II or III endometriosis is not visible at laparoscopy, these lesions are easily missed if the surgeon is not experienced in palpating indurations. In a prospective study of women with infertility and/or pelvic pain a routine clinical examination demonstrated an induration in four out of 58 women whereas during menstruation painful nodularities were felt in 22. These nodularities subsequently proved to be deep endometriosis and/or cystic endometriosis.

Because of these observations, a clinical examination during menstruation has become a routine procedure at our hospital in all women with pelvic pain and in those scheduled for a diagnostic laparoscopy for pelvic pain and/or infertility. The experience gathered thus far can be summarized as follows. Firstly, in almost all women with painful nodularities felt by clinical examination during menstruation, pathology was found during subsequent laparoscopy, suggesting a specificity of almost 100%, even if done by junior and inexperienced registrars. Secondly, a series of women have been operated for deep endometriosis who would otherwise not even have had a diagnostic laparoscopy. It is difficult to estimate the impact of the menstrual clinical examination upon diagnostic accuracy during laparoscopy, i.e. the number of women in whom the diagnosis would have been missed at laparoscopy without a menstrual clinical examination, since this would require a prospective study with a blinded surgeon. However, a series of women in whom no endometriosis had been found at first operation have, since the introduction of the menstrual clinical examination, been reoperated and deep lesions have been excised. The impact of a menstrual clinical examination for

the diagnosis of deep endometriosis is anticipated to be even more important when the surgeon is less experienced with deep lesions. Thirdly, a menstrual clinical examination has demonstrated that in some women deep lesions can be vary small and much more frequent than was thought until recently and that the very small lesions are sometimes apparent during the beginning of the menstrual cycle only. If surgery is performed at the end of the cycle and/or if these women are given a medical pretreatment for endometriosis, many of these lesions are easily missed. Therefore, since deep endometriosis is so strongly associated with pelvic pain, a menstrual clinical examination should be performed in all women with chronic pelvic pain, severe dysmenorrhea and/or deep dyspareunia.

Plasma CA125 concentrations can help to diagnose deep endometriosis (Koninckx, 1993; Koninckx *et al.*, 1996). We reported that, using a cut-off limit of 35 U/ml, the diagnosis of deep endometriosis could be made with an overall sensitivity of 36% and a specificity of 87%. However, taking into account that mainly type III lesions are difficult to diagnose and that these are the most deeply situated lesions which secrete preferentially to the peripheral circulation (Koninckx *et al.*, 1992), the real clinical usefulness of CA125 assays is much better. Since CA125 concentrations in endometriosis are specifically increased during menstruation (Pittaway and Fayez, 1987; O'Shaughnessy, 1993) we postulated that the diagnostic accuracy could be improved by appropriate sampling during the menstrual cycle. This, however, could not be substantiated since in women with endometriotic disease, continuously elevated concentrations of CA125 are found. The highest diagnostic accuracy is obtained during the mid-follicular phase and these CA125 concentrations, together with a menstrual clinical examination, can be used with a sensitivity and specificity of nearly 100% to diagnose deep endometriosis or at least to decide to whom a bowel preparation should be given.

Diagnosis cannot be made by abdominal and vaginal ultrasound examination or by nuclear magnetic resonance imaging (Deprest *et al.*, 1993; Koninckx *et al.*, 1993). The latter can diagnose most of the severe deep endometriotic lesions, but its diagnostic accuracy is insufficient to be used as a diagnostic tool. Indeed, the presence of smaller deep lesions could not be reliably diagnosed and the lateral spread of the nodule could not be evaluated with sufficient precision to be helpful during surgery.

In conclusion, the diagnosis of deep endometriosis, while being obvious in most women, is probably frequently missed in smaller lesions. Clinical examination during menstruation and plasma CA125 concentrations are currently the most reliable methods to alert one to the diagnosis, which is finally made during excision. It cannot be denied that many women with chronic pelvic pain and/or severe dysmenorrhea, without obvious pathology, in fact have deep endometriosis which will not be diagnosed unless a menstrual clinical examination is performed.

TREATMENT OF DEEP ENDOMETRIOSIS

SURGERY

Surgery is the obvious treatment for deep endometriosis, since the final diagnosis – the depth of infiltration – can only be made during excision. With clinical examination and laparoscopic inspection, the diagnosis can only be suspected. The full depth of infiltration and the shape of the nodule becomes apparent only during excision, i.e. when the surgeon remains carefully at the border between healthy tissue and the endometriotic nodule. It is obvious that neither the depth of infiltration and lateral spread, nor the infiltration in the bowel can be judged adequately by clinical examination or laparoscopic inspection or preoperative ultrasound or MRI examination. Thus a preoperative contrast enema, intravenous pyelogram and careful examination of the posterior fornix are recommended in all women before starting surgery. Moreover, a complete bowel preparation is mandatory in all women suspected of having deep endometriosis since the real extent of disease and bowel infiltration will become apparent only during surgery.

Several surgical techniques have been described: laparoscopy contrasted with laparotomy and CO_2 laser excision with sharp dissection. Vaginal excision, aided by laparoscopy, and partial rectum resection and reanastomosis have been described (Martin and Vander Zwagg, 1987; Davis and Brooks, 1988; Martin, 1988; Mage *et al.*, 1989; Koninckx *et al.*, 1991, 1993; Candiani *et al.*, 1992; Nezhat *et al.*, 1992; Redwine, 1992; Wood *et al.*, 1993; Donnez *et al.*, 1995). Randomized trials are lacking, however, and are almost impossible to perform since few surgeons have the skill and expertise to use several techniques. Since excision of deep endometriosis is, moreover, technically difficult it is obvious that each surgeon prefers the method which he believes is the best and which he has the greatest expertise with. This method undoubtedly is the best method in his hands.

Although smaller lesions can be excised by electrosurgery and scissors, we prefer to use a CO_2 laser together with a high flow insufflator (Koninckx and Vandermeersch, 1991), a three-puncture technique (one 12 mm and two 5 mm trocars) and an operative endoscope with a 7 mm operating channel (Storz, Tüttlingen, Germany). The insufflator permits excision of endometriotic lesions with a continuous laser beam (15 watt Superpulse, Sharplan 1080, Tel Aviv) without visible smoke. Excision is guided visually, endometriosis glowing yellowish under the laser beam, and helped by feeling the indurations, for example with the irrigation cannula. Care is taken to remain at the border between the endometriotic nodule and normal healthy tissue. Although it can occasionally be difficult to distinguish endometriosis from normal tissue, especially when endometriosis is close to the cervix, the difference between the harder nodule and the soft tissue of the pelvis is generally apparent. Complete excision implies that endometriosis has to be resected from the rectum wall which will occasionally be opened, that dissection of the rectovaginal septum has sometimes to be performed up to 3–4 cm below the posterior vaginal fornix which sometimes has to be excised and that endometriosis has eventually to be resected from around the ureter and the uterine artery. This can be especially difficult, since endometriosis has a tendency to infiltrate specifically along the uterine artery. Therefore in severe cases, at the end of surgery both ureters should always be identified and 120 ml of air should be introduced into the rectum with 1 liter of fluid in the pouch of Douglas, in order not to miss unnoticed bowel injuries.

Since the depth and the lateral spread of the endometriosis cannot be evaluated before surgery, a complete bowel preparation should be given in order to permit a complete excision. In women with larger lesions a preoperative contrast barium enema, an intravenous pyelogram and colonoscopy should be performed. If gross distortion of the ureter is present, preoperative ureteric stents are recommended. When part of the rectal wall has to be removed or when the rectum is accidentally opened, the pelvis is rinsed with a 1% Hibitane solution and the wall is sutured endoscopically with two layers of 3-0 Vicryl (Ethicon, USA). A defect in the posterior vaginal fornix is sutured either vaginally or endoscopically. Care is taken to suture these defects so that they are water-tight and we prefer to suture them laparoscopically, for reasons of sterility. During laparoscopic suturing a continuous flow of CO_2 from the abdominal cavity to the vagina prevents contamination.

Surgical excision of deep endometriosis is difficult since it often necessitates dissection laterally around the ureter and uterine artery. Also the excision from the bowel wall is difficult, since in 10% of women part of the bowel wall will have to be resected. In 20% of women, especially those with rectovaginal endometriosis, i.e. type III lesions, excision has to be performed up to and including the posterior vaginal fornix. Neither resection of part of the bowel wall nor resection of the vaginal fornix should be considered as complications of surgery, since the postoperative follow-up has been uneventful in a series of over 300 women.

Complications of surgery (n = 225) have been the transsection of the uterine artery in two women, necessitating clipping, a ureteric lesion in one woman and a late bowel perforation in six women. A ureteric lesion is a serious complication and therefore we advocate a preoperative intravenous pyelogram, a careful dissection of the ureter from its landmarks at the pelvic brim and liberal preventive stenting if necessary. This is judged even more important since we realized that a ureter which is only half cut can be sutured endoscopically over a double J (Neven *et al.*, 1993). A late bowel perforation is an even more serious complication which has occurred in six women: two women with a type II lesion and one woman with a type III lesion were readmitted after a week with progressively increasing symptoms of peritonitis; one woman with a type I lesion and a history of pouch anastomosis for colitis ulcerosa was observed for one week with atypical symptoms which later proved to be a rectal perforation. Two women with a type II lesion had acute pelvic pain 12 hours following surgery and two days following surgery respectively. Although symptoms of peritonitis were minimal, an immediate laparoscopy revealed a bowel perforation in both.

It is important to realize that bowel perforations can occur during the first postoperative days, thus necessitating a low fiber diet and eventually hospitalization. A perforation generally occurs during straining, with acute pelvic pain as the only symptom. Disturbingly, this pain disappears over the next few hours with slight peritoneal irritation as the only symptom. A liberal use of early second-look laparoscopy is advocated in these women before symptoms of peritonitis develop. In two women we recently demonstrated that even a bowel perforation can safely be sutured endoscopically, thus avoiding a colostomy.

In conclusion, surgical excision of deep endometriosis can be performed endoscopically provided the necessary training has been provided and experience acquired. It requires routine dissection of the ureter and uterine artery and bowel surgery. Occasionally even ureteric surgery might be necessary. In order to prevent late perforations, prophylactic suturing is advocated. Since this is performed liberally, late perforations have virtually disappeared in our series.

MEDICAL TREATMENT

Medical therapy *before surgery* has been discussed for many years and surgeons have claimed that deep lesions were less vascularized following medical therapy. Recently we demonstrated that pretreatment for three months with an LH-RH agonist could shrink the volume of deep lesions (Koninckx *et al.*, 1997). Indeed, in our series decapeptyl (3.75 mg/month) has been given specifically to women with the most severe disease, especially deep lesions. Analysis of data showed that women pretreated with this LH-RH agonist had a much higher rAFS score at surgery than those without treatment, confirming the selection bias. Similarly, pretreated women had more and larger cystic ovarian endometriosis, also pointing to the selection bias. As expected, women with pretreatment had a smaller pelvic area of endometriosis and also a smaller volume of deep endometriosis, notwithstanding the fact that because of the selection bias, they must have had a much higher volume before treatment. For this reason we strongly advocate the pretreatment of women with severe deep endometriosis medically for three months with an LH-RH agonist. We believe that danazol might be equally effective but our series was too small to prove

this statistically. Other medical therapies have not been used frequently enough to be evaluated.

Medical treatment *following* excision of deep endometriosis has not been evaluated properly. If excision has been performed completely, medical treatment is probably not necessary. However, it should be considered instead of repeat or more radical surgery for recurring symptoms or failures of excision.

Medical treatment alone has not been addressed specifically in any study because of the lack of a clearcut diagnosis of deep endometriosis without excision. Medical treatment with danazol, gonadotropin-releasing hormone agonists or gestrinone has been addressed in a large number of excellent studies (Buttram *et al.*, 1985; Hull *et al.*, 1987; Telimaa *et al.*, 1987; Henzl, 1988; Henzl *et al.*, 1988; Cooke and Thomas, 1989; Dmowski *et al.*, 1989; Donnez *et al.*, 1989; Fedele *et al.*, 1989b; Chong *et al.*, 1990; Dlugi *et al.*, 1990; Kennedy *et al.*, 1990; Rolland and van der Heijden, 1990; Trabant *et al.*, 1990; Mettler *et al.*, 1991; Anon, 1992; Dicker *et al.*, 1992; Eldred *et al.*, 1992; Franssen *et al.*, 1992; Reichel *et al.*, 1992; Shaw, 1992; Wheeler *et al.*, 1992, 1993; Rock *et al.*, 1993; Ruiz-Velasco *et al.*, 1993; Vercellini *et al.*, 1993; Adamson *et al.*, 1994; Marcus and Edwards, 1994). Medical therapy decreased the size and number of implants and thus the rAFS score (Fedele *et al.*, 1989a,b, 1993; Shaw, 1990; Redwine *et al.*, 1992) but does not cure endometriosis. It inactivates the endometriotic lesions, which reappear rapidly after treatment has been stopped (Shaw, 1993). None of these therapies has an important beneficial effect on subsequent fertility (Hughes *et al.*, 1993). They all improve pelvic pain and the effect persists often for many months after therapy has been stopped (Buttram, 1993; Adamson *et al.*, 1994). Since deep endometriosis is strongly associated with pelvic pain and since cystic ovarian endometriosis does not respond well to medical therapy, it is suggested that the observations and conclusions concerning severe pelvic pain are probably related to deep endometriosis.

RESULTS OF TREATMENT

FERTILITY

Nehzat *et al.* (1992) reported 25 pregnancies in 67 women following excision of deep endometriosis. We evaluated cumulative pregnancy rates (CPR) in a consecutive series of 900 women with primary or secondary infertility without severe tubal damage and with a severely subfertile husband. Cumulative pregnancy rates were slightly lower in advanced stages of endometriosis according to the revised AFS classification, being 62% and 44% in classes I and IV respectively. However, when the duration of infertility was taken into account – which was the strongest predictor of subsequent conception – the differences in CPR between classes I and IV disappeared, suggesting that the differences found between mild and severe endometriosis were mainly a consequence of differences in duration of infertility and possibly in age of the women.

The only single group with a significantly higher CPR following surgery were women with deep endometriosis. By Cox multivariate regression analysis, the following model was established: pregnancy was predicted most strongly by a shorter duration of infertility and by the surgical treatment of cystic ovarian endometriosis and/or of deep endometriosis. From these results it can be concluded that aggressive and complete excision of deep endometriosis can be advocated, with subsequent spontaneous pregnancy rates up to 60% within one year. These results can be considered excellent taking into account the severity of disease and the large denuded area in the pelvis following excision of deep endometriosis. It remains unclear whether those women who do not conceive after one year should be oriented towards *in vitro* fertilization or to a second-look laparoscopy.

Medical treatment alone, as can be derived from indirect evidence, is probably not the treatment of choice for deep endometriosis and infertility. Medical pretreatment seems to be useful to facilitate surgery, as has been suggested for cystic ovarian endometriosis (Evers, 1987).

PELVIC PAIN

Both surgical and medical treatment were reported to be highly successful in treating pelvic pain. Candiani *et al.* (1992) reported absence of dyspareunia and dysmenorrhea in six and four women respectively out of ten after 40 months. Nezhat *et al.* (1992) reported moderate to complete pain relief in 162 women out of 175 but in some two or more interventions had been necessary. Preliminary analysis of our results in 250 women in whom deep endometriosis has been excised with a CO_2 laser showed a cure rate of pelvic pain in 70% with a recurrence rate of less than 5% with a follow-up period of up to five years. These data should be interpreted carefully, since the completeness of excision has steadily increased. The results of the latter years strongly suggest an almost complete cure rate without recurrences; this, however, could be an overoptimistic clinical impression which will have to be proven by careful analysis of the data. Also, medical treatment of pelvic pain is highly efficient and the effect of treatment often persists after treatment has been stopped (Buttram, 1993).

CONCLUSIONS AND DISCUSSION

Diagnosis of deep endometriosis is still a clinical problem. Pelvic tenderness at clinical examination and laparoscopy remain the cornerstones of diagnosis, which can be helped by elevated CA125 concentration in plasma and a pelvic examination during menstruation. However, the impression persists that smaller lesions, which are sometimes discovered 'by accident' during endoscopic surgery, frequently remain undiagnosed and that some 'normal' women with chronic pelvic pain might harbor small deep endometriotic nodules.

The choice of treatment will depend upon the local expertise and invasiveness of surgery. If surgery can be performed during the diagnostic laparoscopy by endoscopic surgery, this is probably the method of choice. Indeed, hospitalization and morbidity are only slightly higher than with diagnostic laparoscopy alone and results are excellent. This approach, however, requires a full preoperative investigation of bowel and ureter, whereas a medical pretreatment is suggested in women with severe disease. If more invasive surgery is performed during a second intervention, the advantages and disadvantages of surgical and medical therapy should be balanced, taking into account the excellent results of medical therapy upon pelvic pain. If a first surgery has been incomplete and pain symptoms recur, medical treatment seems to be the preferred treatment.

ACKNOWLEDGMENTS

We thank our co-workers and co-authors of articles from which data have been taken. Stefan Lempereur MD, Ipsen NV, Belgium, and Freddy Cornillie PhD, Director Centocor Europe, are thanked for their support and co-operation. This work was supported partially by the NFWO research grant number 9-002090.

REFERENCES

Adamson, G.D., Kwei, L. and Edgren, R.A. (1994) Pain of endometriosis: effects of nafarelin and danazol therapy. *Int J Fertil Menopausal Stud*, **39**, 215–17.

Andrews, W.C., Buttram, V.C.J., Behrman, S.J. *et al.* (1985) Revised American Fertility Society classification of endometriosis. *Fertil Steril*, **44**, 7–8.

Anonymous (1992) Nafarelin for endometriosis: a large-scale, danazol-controlled trial of efficacy and safety, with 1-year follow-up. The Nafarelin European Endometriosis Trial Group (NEET) [see comments]. *Fertil Steril*, **57**, 514–22.

Ayers, J.W.T. and Friedenstab, A.P. (1985) *Utero-Tubal Hypotonia Associated with Pelvic Endometriosis.* Proceedings of the 41st American Fertility Society meeting (abstract).

Badawy, S.Z.A., Cuenca, V., Marshall, L. *et al.* (1984) Cellular components in peritoneal fluid in infertile patients with and without endometriosis. *Fertil Steril*, **42**, 704–8.

Bartosik, D., Jacobs, S.L. and Kelly, L.J. (1986) Endometrial tissue in peritoneal fluid. *Fertil Steril*, **46**, 796–800.

Buttram, V.C. (1993) Rationale for combined medical and surgical treatment of endometriosis, in *The Current State of Endometriosis*, (eds. I.A. Brosens and J. Donnez), Parthenon Publishing, New York, pp. 320–406.

Buttram, V.C.J., Reiter, R.C. and Ward, S. (1985) Treatment of endometriosis with danazol: report of a 6-year prospective study. *Fertil Steril*, **44**, 36–43.

Candiani, G.B., Vercelline, P., Fedele, L. *et al.* (1992) Conservative surgical treatment of rectovaginal septum endometriosis. *J Gynecol Surg*, **8**, 177–82.

Chong, A.P., Keene, M.E. and Thornoton, N.L. (1989) Comparison of three modes of treatment for infertility patients with minimal pelvic endometriosis. *Fertil Steril*, **53**, 407–10.

Cooke, L.D. and Thomas, E.J. (1989) The medical treatment of mild endometriosis. *Acta Obstet Gynecol Scand* (suppl), 27–30.

Cornillie, F.J., Oosteerlynck, D., Lauweryns, J.M. and Koninckx, P.R. (1990) Deeply infiltrating pelvic endometriosis: histology and clinical significance. *Fertil Steril*, **53**, 978–83.

Cullen, T.S. (1986a) Adenoma-myoma uteri diffusum benignum. *Johns Hopkins Hosp Bull*, **6**, 133–7.

Cullen, T.S. (1986b) Adeno-myoma of the round ligament. *Johns Hopkins Hosp Bull*, **7**, 112–14.

Davis, G.D. and Brooks, R.A. (1988) Excision of pelvic endometriosis with the carbon dioxide laser laparoscope. *Obstet Gynecol*, **72**, 816–19.

Deprest, J., Marchal, G. and Koninckx, P.R. (1993) *MRI in the Diagnosis of Deeply Infiltrating Endometriosis.* Proceedings of the AAGl 22nd annual meeting (abstract).

D'Hooghe, T.M., Barmbra, C.S., Cornillie, F.J. *et al.* (1991) Prevalence and laparoscopic appearance of spontaneous endometriosis in the baboon (*Papio anubis, Papio cynocephalus*). *Biol Reprod*, **45**, 411–16.

D'Hooghe, T.M., Bambra, C.S., Isahakia, M. and Koninckx, P.R. (1992) Evolution of spontaneous endometriosis in the baboon (*Papio anubis, Papio cynocephalus*) over a 12-month period. *Fertil Steril*, **58**, 409–12.

D'Hooghe, T.M., Bambra, C.S., Suleman, M.A., Dunselman, G.A., Evers, H.L. and Koninckx, P.R. (1994) Development of a model of retrograde menstruation in baboons (*Papio anubis*). *Fertil Steril*, **62**, 635–8.

D'Hooghe, T.M., Bambra, C.S., Raeymaekers, B.M. *et al.* (1995) Intrapelvic injection of menstrual endometrium causes endometriosis in baboons (*Papio cynocephalus* and *Papio anubis*). *Am J Obstet Gynceol*, **173**, 125–34.

Dicker, D., Goldman, J.A., Levy, T. *et al.* (1992) The impact of long-term gonadotropin-releasing hormone analogue treatment on preclinical abortions in patients with severe endometriosis undergoing in vitro fertilization-embryo transfer. *Fertil Steril*, **57**, 579–600.

Dlugi, A.M., Miller, J.D. and Knittle, J. (1990) Lupron depot (leuprolide acetate for depot suspension) in the treatment of endometriosis: a randomized, placebo-controlled, double-blind study. *Fertil Steril*, **54**, 419–27.

Dmowski, W.P., Steele, R.W. and Baker, G.F. (1981) Deficient cellular immunity in endometriosis. *Am J Obstet Gynceol*, **141**, 377–83.

Dmowski, W.P., Radwanska, E., Binor, Z. *et al.* (1989) Ovarian suppression induced with buserelin or danazol in the management of endometriosis: a randomized, comparative study. *Fertil Steril*, **51**, 395–400.

Donnez, J., Nisolle, M., Clerckx Braun, F. *et al.* (1989) Administration of nasal Buserelin as compared with subcutaneous Buserelin implant for endometriosis. *Fertil Steril*, **52**, 27–30.

Donnez, J., Nisolle, M., Casanasroux, F. *et al.* (1995) Rectovaginal septum, endometriosis or adenomyosis: laparoscopic management in a series of 231 patients. *Human Reprod*, **10**, 630–5.

Eisermann, J., Gast, M.J., Pineda, J. *et al.* (1988) Tumor necrosis factor in peritoneal fluid of women undergoing laparoscopic surgery. *Fertil Steril*, **50**, 573–9.

Eldred, J.M., Haynes, P.J. and Thomas, E.J. (1992) A randomized double-blind placebo-controlled trial of the effects on bone metabolism of the combination of nafarelin acetate and norethisterone. *Clin Endocrinol*, **37**, 354–9.

El Mahgoub, S. and Yaseen, S. (1980) A positive proof for the theory of coelomic metaplasia. *Am J Obstet Gynecol*, **137**, 173–40.

Evers, J.L.H. (1987) The second-look laparoscopy for evaluation of the result of medical treatment of endometriosis should not be performed during ovarian suppression. *Fertil Steril*, **47**, 502–4.

Evers, J.L. (1989) The pregnancy rate of the no-treatment group in randomized clinical trials of endometriosis therapy. *Fertil Steril*, **52**, 906–7.

Evers, J.L.H. (1993) The immune system in endometriosis: introduction, in *The Current Status of Endometriosis*, (eds. I.A. Brosens and J. Donnez), Parthenon Publishing, New York, pp. 223–33.

Fakih, H., Bagett, B., Holtz, G. *et al.* (1987) Interleukin-1: a possible role in the infertility associated with endometriosis. *Fertil Steril*, **47**, 213–700.

Fedele, L., Arcaini, L., Bianchi, S. *et al.* (1989a) Comparison of cyproterone acetate and danazol in the treatment of pelvic pain associated with endometriosis. *Obstet Gynecol*, **73**, 1000–4.

Fedele, L., Bianchi, S., Arcaini, L. *et al.* (1989b) Buserelin versus danazol in the treatment of endometriosis-associated infertility. *Am J Obstet Gynecol*, **161**, 871–6.

Fedele, L., Bianchi, S., Bocciolone, L. *et al.* (1993) Buserelin acetate in the treatment of pelvic pain associated with minimal and mild endometriosis – a controlled study. *Fertil Steril*, **59**, 516–21.

Franssen, A.M.H.W., van der Heijden, P.F.M., Thomas, C.M.G. *et al.* (1992) On the origin and significance of serum CA-125 concentrations in 97 patients with endometriosis before, during and after buserelin acetate, nafarelin, or danazol. *Fertil Steril*, **57**, 974–9.

Halme, J. (1989) Release of tumor necrosis factor-alpha by human peritoneal macrophages in vivo and in vitro. *Am J Obstet Gynecol*, **161**, 1718–25.

Halme, J., Becker, S. and Haskill, S. (1987) Altered maturation and function of peritoneal macrophages: possible role in pathogenesis of endometriosis. *Am J Obstet Gynecol*, **156**, 783–9.

Haney, A.F. (1993) Endometriosis, macrophages, and adhesions. *Prog Clin Biol Res*, **381**, 19–44.

Haney, A.F. and Weinberg, J.B. (1988) Reduction of the intraperitoneal inflammation associated with endometriosis by treatment with medroxyprogesterone acetate. *Am J Obstet Gynecol*, **159**, 450–4.

Haney, A.F., Muscato, J.J. and Weinberg, J.B. (1981) Peritoneal fluid cell populations in infertility patients. *Fertil Steril*, **35**, 696–8.

Henzl, M.R. (1988) Gonadotropin-releasing hormone (GnRH) agonists in the management of endometriosis: a review. *Clin Obstet Gynecol*, **31**, 840–56.

Henzi, M.R., Corson, S.L., Moghissi, K. *et al.* (1988) Administration of nasal nafarelin as compared with oral danazol for endometriosis. A multicenter double-blind comparative clinical trial. *N Engl J Med*, **318**, 485–9.

Hoshiai, H., Ishikawa, M., Sawatari, Y. *et al.* (1993) Laparoscopic evaluation of the onset and progression of endometriosis. *Am J Obstet Gynecol*, **169**, 714–19.

Hughes, E.G., Fedorkow, D.M. and Collins, J.A. (1993) A quantitative overview of controlled trials in endometriosis-associated infertility. *Fertil Steril*, **59**, 963–70.

Hull, M.E., Moghissi, K.S. *et al.* (1987) Comparison of different treatment modalities of endometriosis in infertile women. *Fertil Steril*, **47**, 40–4.

Jansen, R.P.S. and Russel, P. (1986) Nonpigmented endometriosis: clinical, laparoscopic, and pathologic definition. *Am J Obstet Gynecol*, **155**, 1154–9.

Jenkins, S., Olive, D.L. and Haney, A.F. (1986) Endometriosis: pathogenetic implications of the anatomic distribution. *Obstet Gynecol*, **67**, 335–8.

Kennedy, S.H., Williams, I.A., Brodribb, J. *et al.* (1990) A comparison of nafarelin acetate and danazol in the treatment of endometriosis. *Fertil Steril*, **53**, 998–1003.

Koninckx, P.R. (1993) CA-125 in the management of endometriosis. *Eur J Obstet Gynecol Reprod Biol*, **49**, 109–13.

Koninckx, P.R. (1994a) Is mild endometriosis a condition occurring intermittently in all women? *Human Reprod*, **9**, 2202–5.

Koninckx, P.R. (1994b) The growth and development of endometriosis, in *Growth and Differentiation in Reproductive Organs*, (eds. A.R. Genazzai, F. Petraglia, A.D. Genazzani and G. D'Ambrogio), CIC Editzionii International, Roma, pp. 272–9.

Koninckx, P.R. (1995) Diagnostic et traitement de l'endometriose profonde. *References*, **3**, 205–20.

Koninckx, P.R. and Brosens, I.A. (1977) *Diagnosis of the Luteinized Unruptured Follicle Syndrome*. Proceedings of FIGO, Tokyo (abstract).

Koninckx, P.R. and Martin, D.C. (1992) Deep endometriosis: a consequence of infiltration or retraction or possibly adenomyosis externa? *Fertil Steril*, **58**, 924–8.

Koninckx, P.R. and Martin, D. (1994) Treatment of deeply infiltrating endometriosis. *Curr Opin Obstet Gynecol*, **6**, 231–41

Koninckx, P.R. and Martin, D.C. (1995) Surgical treatment of deeply infiltrating endometriosis, in *Endometriosis. Current Understanding and Manage-*

ment, 1st edn, (ed. R.W. Shaw), Blackwell Scientific, Oxford, pp. 264–81.

Koninckx, P.R. and Vandermeersch, E. (1991) The persufflator: an insufflation device for laparoscopy and especially for CO-2-laser-endoscopic surgery. *Human Reprod*, **6**, 1288–90.

Koninckx, P.R., Ide, P., Vandenbroucke, W. and Brosens, I.A. (1980a) New aspects of the pathophysiology of endometriosis and associated infertility. *J Reprod Med*, **24**, 257–60.

Koninckx, P.R., de Moor, P. and Brosens, I.A. (1980b) Diagnosis of the luteinized unruptured follicle syndrome by steroid hormone assays on peritoneal fluid. *Br J Obstet Gynaecol*, **87**, 929–34.

Koninckx, P.R., Heyns, W., Verhoeven, G. *et al.* (1980c) Biochemical characterisation of peritoneal fluid in women during the menstrual cycle. *J Clin Endocrinol Metab*, **51**, 1239–44.

Koninckx, P.R., Meuleman, C., Demeyere, S. *et al.* (1991) Suggestive evidence that pelvic endometriosis is a progressive disease, whereas deeply infiltrating endometriosis is associated with pelvic pain. *Fertil Steril*, **55**, 759–65.

Koninckx, P.R., Riittinen, L., Seppala, M. and Cornillie, F.J. (1992) CA-125 and placental protein 14 concentrations in plasma and peritoneal fluid of women with deeply infiltrating pelvic endometriosis. *Fertil Steril*, **57**, 523–30.

Koninckx, P.R., Deprest, J., Meuleman, C. and Martin, D.C. (1993) The method of destruction of endometriosis makes a difference. *Fertil Steril*, **60**, 202–3.

Koninckx, P.R., Oosterlynck, D., D'Hooghe, T. and Meuleman, C. (1994) Deeply infiltrating endometriosis is a disease whereas mild endometriosis could be considered a non-disease. *Ann NY Acad Sci*, **734**, 333–41.

Koninckx, P.R., Meuleman, C., Oosterlynck, D. and Cornillie, F.J. (1996) Diagnosis of deep endometriosis by clinical examination during menstruation and plasma CA-125 concentration. *Fertil Steril*, **65**, 280–7.

Koninckx, P.R. *et al.* (1997) Complications of surgical excision of deep endometriosis. *Human Reprod*, in press.

Kruitwagen, R.F.P.M., Poels, L.G., Willemsen, W.N.P. *et al.* (1991) Endometrial epithelial cells in peritoneal fluid during the early follicular phase. *Fertil Steril*, **55**, 297–303.

Mage, G., Canis, M., Manhes, H. *et al.* (1989) Laparoscopic treatment of endometriosis. *Contracept Fertil Sex*, **17**, 347–52.

Marcus, S.F. and Edwards, R.G. (1994) High rates of pregnancy after long-term down-regulation of women with severe endometriosis. *Am J Obstet Gynecol*, **171**, 812–17.

Martin, D.C. (1988) Laparoscopic and vaginal colpotomy for the excision of infiltrating cul-de-sac endometriosis. *J Reprod Med Obstet Gynecol*, **33**, 806–8.

Martin, D.C. and Vander Zwagg, R. (1987) Excisional techniques for endometriosis with the CO-2 laser laparoscope. *J Reprod Med*, **32**, 753–8.

Martin, D.C., Hubert, G.D. and Levy, B.S. (1989a) Depth of infiltration of endometriosis. *J Gynecol Surg*, **5**, 55–60.

Martin, D.C., Hubert, G.D., Vander Zwagg, R. and El Zeky, F.A. (1989b) Laparoscopic appearances of peritoneal endometriosis. *Fertil Steril*, **51**, 63–7.

Martin, D.C., Ahmic, R., El Zeky, F.A. *et al.* (1990) Increased histologic confirmation of endometriosis. *J Gynecol Surg*, **6**, 2755–9.

Mettler, L., Steinmuller, H. and Schachner Wunschmann, E. (1991) Experience with a depot GnRH-agonist (Zoladex) in the treatment of genital endometriosis. *Human Reprod*, **6**, 694–8.

Murphy, A.A., Green, W.R., Bobbie, D. *et al.* (1986) Unsuspected endometriosis documented by scanning electron microscopy in visually normal peritoneum. *Fertil Steril*, **46**, 522–4.

Neven, P., Vandeursen, H., Baert, L. and Koninckx, P.R. (1993) Ureteric injury at laparoscopic surgery: the endoscopic management. Case review. *Gynecol Endosc*, **2**, 45–6.

Nezhat, C., Nezhat, F. and Pennington, E. (1992) Laparoscopic treatment of infiltrative rectosigmoid colon and rectovaginal septum endometriosis by the technique of videolaparoscopy and the CO-2 laser. *Br J Obstet Gynaecol*, **99**, 664–7.

Olive, D.L., Weinberg, J.B. and Haney, A.F. (1985) Peritoneal macrophages and infertility: the association between cell number and pelvic pathology. *Fertil Steril*, **44**, 772–7.

Oosterlynck, D.J., Cornillie, F.J., Waer, M. *et al.* (1991) Women with endometriosis show a defect in natural killer activity resulting in a decreased cytotoxicity to autologous endometrium. *Fertil Steril*, **56**, 45–51.

Oosterlynck, D.J., Meulman, C., Waer, M. *et al.* (1992) The natural killer activity of peritoneal fluid lymphocytes is decreased in women with endometriosis. *Fertil Steril*, **58**, 290–5.

Oosterlynck, D.J., Meuleman, C., Sobis, H. *et al.* (1993) Angiogenic activity of peritoneal fluid from women with endometriosis. *Fertil Steril*, **59**, 778–82.

O'Shaughnessy, A. (1993) CA-125 levels measured in different phases of the menstrual cycle in screening for endometriosis. *Obstet Gynecol*, **81**, 99–103.

Pittaway, D.E. and Fayez, J.A. (1987) Serum CA-125 antigen levels increase during menses. *Am J Obstet Gynecol*, **156**, 75–6.

Redwine, D.B. (1987) Age-related evolution in color appearance of endometriosis. *Fertil Steril*, **48**, 1062–3.

Redwine, D.B. (1992) Laparoscopic en bloc resection for treatment of the obliterated cul-de-sac in endometriosis. *J Reprod Med*, **37**, 695–8.

Redwine, D.B., Elstein, M., Shaw, R. *et al.* (1992) Nafarelin versus danazol versus surgery. *Fertil Steril*, **58**, 455–6.

Reichel, R.P., Schweppe, K., Mettler, L. *et al.* (1992) Goserelin (Zoladex) depot in the treatment of endometriosis. *Fertil Steril*, **57**, 1197–202.

Ripps, B.A. and Martin, D.C. (1991) Focal pelvic tenderness, pelvic pain and dysmenorrhea in endometriosis. *J Reprod Med Obstet Gynecol*, **36**, 470–2.

Rock, J.A., Truglia, J.A. and Caplan, R.J (1993) Zoladex (goserelin acetate implant) in the treatment of endometriosis: a randomized comparison with danazol. The Zoladex Endometriosis Study Group. *Obstet Gynecol*, **82**, 8–205.

Rolland, R. and van der Heijden, P.F.M. (1990) Nafarelin versus danazol in the treatment of endometriosis. *Am J Obstet Gynecol*, **162**, 586–8.

Ruiz-Velasco, V., Arceo J.R. and Armesto, A. (1993) Comparative efficacy of gestrinone and danazol in infertile women with endometriosis. *Int J Fertil Menopaus Stud*, **38**, 22–7.

Sampson, J.A. (1927) Peritoneal endometriosis due to the menstrual dissemination of endometrial tissue into the peritoneal cavity. *Am J Obstet Gynecol*, **14**, 422–69.

Sampson, J.A. (1940) The development of the implantation theory for the development of endometriosis. *Am J Obstet Gynecol*, **40**, 549–57.

Shaw, R.W. (1990) Nafarelin in the treatment of pelvic pain caused by endometriosis. *Am J Obstet Gynecol*, **162**, 574–6.

Shaw, R.W. (1992) An open randomized comparative study of the effect of goserelin depot and danazol in the treatment of endometriosis. *Fertil Steril*, **58**, 265–72.

Shaw, R.W. (1993) Endometriosis: current evaluation of management and rationale for medical therapy, in *The Current Status of Endometriosis*, (eds. I.A. Brosens and J. Donnez), Parthenon Publishing, New York, pp. 371–83.

Stripling, M.C., Martin, D.C., Chatman, D.L. *et al.*

(1988) Subtle appearance of pelvic endometriosis. *Fertil Steril*, **49**, 427–31.

Syrop, C.H. and Halme, J. (1987) Cyclic changes of peritoneal fluid parameters in normal and infertile patients. *Obstet Gynecol*, **69**, 416–19.

Telimaa, S., Puolakka, J., Ronnberg, L. and Kauppila, A. (1987) Placebo-controlled comparison of danazol and high-dose medroxyprogesterone acetate in the treatment of endometriosis. *Gynecol Endocrinol*, **1**, 13–23.

Thomas, E.J. and Cooke, I.D. (1987) Successful treatment of asymptomatic endometriosis: does it benefit infertile women? *Br Med J (Clin Res Ed)*, **294**, 1117–19.

Trabant, H., Widdra, W. and de Looze, S. (1990) Efficacy and safety of intranasal buserelin acetate in the treatment of endometriosis: a review of six clinical trials and comparison with danazol. *Prog Clin Biol Res*, **323**, 357–82.

Vercellini, P., Bocciolone, L. and Crosignani, P.G. (1992) Is mild endometriosis always a disease? *Human Reprod*, **7**, 627–9.

Vercellini, P., Trespidi, L., Colombo, A. *et al.* (1993) A gonadotropin-releasing hormone agonist versus a low-dose oral contraceptive for pelvic pain associated with endometriosis. *Fertil Steril*, **60**, 75–9.

Weinberg, J.B., Haney, A.F., Xu, F.J. and Ramakrishnan, S. (1991) Peritoneal fluid and plasma levels of human macrophage colony-stimulating factor in relation to peritoneal fluid macrophage content. *Blood*, **78**, 513–16.

Wheeler, J.M., Knittle, J.D. and Miller, J.D. (1992) Depot leuprolide acetate versus danazol in the treatment of women with symptomatic endometriosis. I. Efficacy results. *Am J Obstet Gynecol*, **167**, 1367–71.

Wheeler, J.M., Knittle, J.D. and Miller, J.D. (1993) Depot leuprolide acetate versus danazol in the treatment of women with symptomatic endometriosis: a multicentre, double-blind randomized clinical trial. II. Assessment of safety. The Lupron Endometriosis Study Group. *Am J Obstet Gynecol*, **169**, 26–33.

Wiegerinck, M.A., van Dop, P.A. and Brosens, I.A. (1993) The staging of peritoneal endometriosis by the type of active lesion in addition to the revised American Fertility Society classification. *Fertil Steril*, **60**, 461–4.

Wood, C., Hill, D. and Maher, P. (1993) Laparoscopic culdotomy. *Aust NZ J Obstet Gynecol*, **33**, 67–70.

COMPLICATIONS OF LAPAROSCOPIC HYSTERECTOMY

4

R. Garry and G. Phillips

INTRODUCTION

The laparoscope provides a new mode of access to the uterus. In performing a hysterectomy, the uterus to be removed remains the same with the same pathology and the same anatomical relationships whatever the method of removal. All operations are associated with complications and laparoscopic procedures are no exception. Some complications of laparoscopic hysterectomy (LH) represent risks inherent to hysterectomy and some are risks peculiar to the particular technique employed.

The benefits of the laparoscopic approach to hysterectomy have been well rehearsed and include clear highly magnified images, less scarring, less post-operative pain, quicker recovery and in some circumstances considerable financial savings. The potential disadvantages of this approach may include restricted access, lack of tactile sensations, two-dimensional imaging and unfamiliar orientation with the consequent risks of unintended surgery, together with the risks associated with the production of a pneumoperitoneum and the introduction of sharp trocars into the abdominal cavity. The main potential complications associated with laparoscopic hysterectomy (LH) are, however, those associated with the use of novel or unfamiliar equipment in the dangerously congested areas deep in the pelvis.

AUDIT OF COMPLICATIONS

When developing a new technique it is essential to audit every aspect of the procedure but special attention must be paid to assessing the morbidity associated with the new approach. One of the great problems in assessing the incidence, nature and severity of complications of LH is that there is no adequate method of reporting or notifying complications. Instead, we rely on voluntary submissions to a great variety of journals.

In dealing with the rate of complications we need to quantify the numerator (i.e. the absolute number of a particular complication) and the denominator (i.e. the total number of operations performed).

PROBLEMS WITH THE NUMERATOR

Should we have statutory rules for notification of complications? When a new drug is introduced it will have undergone a series of statutory trials resulting in a new product with known efficacy and potential short and medium term side effects. The knowledge of longer term side effects relies on statutory postmarketing surveillance.

Surgeons are in the privileged position of being able to introduce new treatments when the surgeon and patient mutually agree on the advisability and suitability of the new treatment. In practice this works very well but

Gynecological Endoscopic Surgery. Edited by C.J.G. Sutton. Published in 1997 by Chapman & Hall, London. ISBN 0 412 58040 3.

without adequate information on the frequency, nature and severity of complications, it will not be possible for patients to give informed consent or for surgeons to advise patients in an objective and scientific manner.

Surgeons may only continue to work and develop new procedures if patients continue to trust in the surgeon's benign and philanthropic nature. It is therefore vital that complications are reported fully and in a widely accessible way. Clearly the organization required for this is not yet available and so we continue to rely on ad hoc reporting in numerous publications, from a large number of countries and surgical associations.

PROBLEMS WITH THE DENOMINATOR

In the United Kingdom it is difficult to know with any degree of confidence how many laparoscopic hysterectomies are being performed because of inaccuracies within 'Hospital Event Statistics' (HES). This is the system through which the Department of Health monitors all hospital activities.

In this system all operations are coded according to Office of Population Censuses and Surveys (OPCS) codes. Unfortunately the codes tend to lag behind the latest developments by many years and this means that operations may easily be miscoded, resulting, for instance, in a laparoscopically assisted vaginal hysterectomy being coded as a vaginal hysterectomy. In addition to this different hospitals may code the same operation in different ways.

These systematic errors are compounded by individual errors and the resultant effect is that figures for complication rates are likely to be extremely inaccurate. Similarly, any comparison between vaginal, abdominal and laparoscopic procedures will be difficult to interpret.

LITERATURE REVIEW

Table 4.1 summarizes the complications gleaned from a search of predominantly Eng-

lish language journals and is not exhaustive. There are a total of 3189 hysterectomies included, from both prospective and retrospective studies (O'Connor *et al.*, personal communication; Garcia-Padial *et al.*, 1992; Grainger *et al.*, 1992; Liu, 1992, 1993a; Nezhat *et al.*, 1992; Summitt *et al.*, 1992; Boike *et al.*, 1993; Bronitsky *et al.*, 1993; Donnez and Nisolle, 1993; Hasson *et al.*, 1993; Houreabie and Bruhat, 1993; Howard and Sanchez, 1993; Hunter and McCartney, 1993; Phipps *et al.*, 1993; Querleu *et al.*, 1993b; Reich *et al.*, 1993; Saye *et al.*, 1993; Schwartz *et al.*, 1993; Arbogast *et al.*, 1994; Bruhat *et al.*, 1994; Casey *et al.*, 1994; Ewen and Sutton, 1994; Mencaglia *et al.*, 1994; Ou *et al.*, 1994; Wood *et al.*, 1994a,b; Garry and Hercz, 1995; Jones, 1995). The definitions and criteria for side effects clearly vary between studies; for instance, many of the reports do not define what is meant by a postoperative fever or the definitions vary. The clarity of the reports also varies and where there is some doubt as to the nature or severity of a complication or its treatment, it has been assumed that the complication was more rather than less severe and that treatment was more rather than less extensive. For instance, the trocar herniae are assumed to have included bowel (where it is not stated) and are therefore counted as bowel injuries requiring laparotomy, unless the treatment is otherwise specified.

Table 4.2 compares the complications with those reported by Dicker *et al.* (1982) for abdominal and vaginal hysterectomy. This is the largest series of prospectively collected data on the complications of these operations and is a reliable basis for comparing the complications of LH. The main criticisms of this series are, firstly, that antibiotics were given infrequently in the abdominal hysterectomy group compared to the vaginal group, which in turn had a much lower febrile morbidity rate; and secondly, the rate of unintended major surgery in the vaginal group seems very high at 5.1%.

Amirikia and Evans (1979) reported compli-

Table 4.1 Complications of 3189 laparoscopic hysterectomies

Complication	Number	%
ALL MAJOR URINARY TRACT INJURIES	**44**	**1.38**
35 bladder and 9 ureter injuries requiring laparotomy or, rarely, laparoscopic repair		
Bladder laceration (recognized at op.)	29	0.91
Ureteric injury (recognized at op.)	4	0.13
Late diagnosed injuries (fistulae: 2 ureterovaginal, 3 vesicovaginal, 2 vesicoabdominal, 2 unspecified) (2 ureteric occlusions – 1 resulted in nephrectomy)	11	0.35
Urinary retention	10	0.31
MAJOR BOWEL INJURY	**15**	**0.47**
Includes 13 traumatic injuries, 1 internal hernia and 1 as a result of a pelvic abscess which resulted in a temporary colostomy		
Small bowel obstruction not requiring operation	6	0.19
ALL TROCAR PROBLEMS	**50**	**1.57**
Includes 2 Veress needle injuries		
Major vessel injury (Veress needle)	2	0.06
Epigastric artery injury	10	0.31
Trocar site hernia	10	0.31
Trocar site bruising/cellulitis/infection	28	0.88
HEMORRHAGE REQUIRING TRANSFUSION	**39**	**1.22**
LAPAROTOMY	**110**	**3.45**
Includes conversion to TAH and repairs to all injuries requiring laparotomy where the treatment is not specified		
Repeat laparoscopy	8	0.25
PULMONARY EMBOLUS	**6**	**0.19**
VAULT PROBLEMS	**35**	**1.10**
Hematoma or bleeding 30, cuff cellulitis 2, peritoneovaginal fistula 1, pelvic abscess or infection 2 – 1 of these required partial colectomy and temporary colostomy		
ALL FEBRILE MORBIDITY	**137**	**4.30**
Includes UTI, pneumonia, unexplained fever, cuff cellulitis, trocar wound infections and cellulitis		
Urinary tract infection	27	0.85
Unexplained fever	43	1.35
Pneumonia/atelectasis	5	0.16
CERVICAL STUMP PROBLEMS	**8**	**0.25**
Continued menses 6, mucorrhea 2 and includes 2 subsequent cervicectomies		
DEATH	**1**	**0.03**
Patient who developed pneumonia then ARDS		
OTHER MINOR COMPLICATIONS	**87**	**2.72**
Hematuria 5, autologous transfusion 30, nerve injury (resolved) 5, subcutaneous emphysema 2, fluid overload 3, arrhythmia 1, knee pain 1, dehydration 1, minor hemorrhage 9, anemia 8, headache/nausea 6, tendinitis 1, pain 2, hematoma ?where 10, transient depression 3		
TOTAL	498	15.62

Table 4.2   Comparison of complication rates of hysterectomy (rate per 100 women undergoing hysterectomy). The rates for vaginal and abdominal hysterectomy are taken from Dicker *et al.* (1982)

Complications (%)	Laparoscopic (n = 3189)	Vaginal (n = 568)	Abdominal (n = 1283)
FEBRILE MORBIDITY	**4.3**	**15.3**	**32.3**
Unexplained	1.3	7.2	16.8
Urinary infection	0.8	3.4	7.0
Abdominal wound infection (includes trocar wound cellulitis and hematoma)	0.9	0	5.0
Vaginal cuff infection (includes vault hematoma)	1.0*	2.1	3.1
Pelvic infection	0.1	1.2	1.3
Upper respiratory tract infection	–	0.9	0.4
Pneumonia	0.2	0.4	0.4
Sepsis	–	0.4	0.2
Peritonitis	–	0.2	0
TRANSFUSION	**1.2**	**8.3**	**15.4**
Not autologous			
UNINTENDED MAJOR SURGERY	**3.5**	**5.1**	**1.7**
Includes conversion to abdominal hysterectomy			
BOWEL TRAUMA	**0.5**	**0.6**	**0.3**
URINARY TRACT TRAUMA	**1.4**	**1.6**	**0.5**
Bladder trauma	1.1	1.6	0.3
Ureteric injury	0.3	0	0.2
PULMONARY EMBOLUS	**0.2**	**0**	**0.2**
OVERALL	**15.6**	**24.5**	**42.8**

Table 4.3   Comparison of complication rates of abdominal and vaginal hysterectomy from Dicker *et al.* (1982) and Amirikia and Evans (1979)

	Vaginal		Abdominal	
	Dicker	*Amirikia*	*Dicker*	*Amirikia*
Fever	15.3	26	32.3	16
Transfusion	8.3	7	15.4	15
Bladder injury	1.6	0.18	0.3	0.4
Ureter injury	0	0.1	0.2	0.11
Bowel injury	0.6	0	0.3	0.2
Pulmonary embolus	0	0.1	0.2	0.34

cations of 6435 hysterectomies carried out between 1965 and 1974 and their complication rates were similar to Dicker's, especially for abdominal hysterectomy. They had a similar proportion of vaginal (33%) and abdominal (66%) hysterectomies, but had a 1% incidence of radical and cesarean hysterectomies. Table 4.3 illustrates their overall complication rates, but unfortunately Amirikia and Evans do not quote a rate for unintended major surgery or laparotomy. Each group of injuries is discussed in the sections that follow.

ACCESS PROBLEMS

OVERVIEW

Conventional vaginal and abdominal hysterectomies have their own access problems. The previously scarred abdominal wall, obesity and intra-abdominal adhesions may all cause difficulty and complications during the abdominal approach to the uterus. Previous surgery and scarring, lack of descent, lack of vaginal width and the tight introitus may result in access problems during the vaginal approach. In all of these cases bowel, vascular and urinary tract injury may arise. What the patient and the surgeon would like to know is whether these complications are more severe and more frequent during the laparoscopic approach to hysterectomy. For the reasons explained above these questions cannot be answered with great accuracy; nevertheless, a slightly broader perspective is required when dealing with complications.

INSTRUMENTS

Inadvertent injuries to intra-abdominal structures are more likely to occur if instruments are blunt or poorly maintained. Blunt trocars and Veress needles require more pressure to insert them and therefore an 'overshoot' injury is more likely to occur. It is one of the surgeon's many responsibilities to ensure that he or she does not continue to use poorly maintained equipment. The theater manager will not know unless told.

The various parts of the Veress needle must fit together correctly so that the central blunt-ended probe protrudes beyond the outer sheath and does move back as the needle is introduced. The spring must be able to push the central blunt probe back out once the needle is in the abdominal cavity. The surgeon must pay attention to these details in the interests of safety.

Trocars with spring-loaded protective safety shields are available from the various manufacturers. It is not clearly established that they give improved safety although the trocar will be sharp every time. Despite this, in Soderstrom's (1993) review of 66 bowel perforations resulting in litigation, disposable trocars with safety shields were used in 12 cases.

The debate on the use of disposable and reusable trocars and needles will continue. Both are safe but how much extra safety can be bought by using disposables is unclear.

VASCULAR INJURY IN THE ABDOMINAL WALL

Blood vessels may be damaged in the anterior abdominal wall or on the posterior wall of the abdomen as a result of direct injury with the Veress needle or with any of the trocars that are used. Occasionally, particularly if there are omental adhesions, vessels lying in the omentum or the gut mesentery may be injured.

Multiple punctures and the use of larger trocars increase the risk of vascular injury. Similarly the obese patient and those with a previous Pfannenstiel incision may have distorted anatomy in the anterior abdominal wall so that anatomical landmarks may be lost and transillumination, when it is used, may be unhelpful. It is important to recognize these risk factors and place the lateral trocars accordingly.

Inferior epigastric vessels

These vessels lie deep in the anterior abdominal wall between the rectus muscle and the peritoneum. The artery usually lies lateral to the obliterated umbilical artery and runs just under the lateral edge of the rectus muscles and is accompanied by two venae commitantes between which it lies. It arises from the external iliac artery and eventually anastomoses with the superior epigastric artery. Only in the slimmest of patients will it be possible to transilluminate these vessels as they lie so deep.

Laceration of the inferior epigastrics will therefore tend to produce intraperitoneal bleeding or bleeding into the potential space between the recti and the peritoneum. Large amounts of blood may be lost and large hematomata produced, with significant morbidity.

It is absolutely essential to use a sound method for avoiding these vessels. Trocars must *always* be inserted under direct laparoscopic vision and perpendicular to the skin to minimize the thickness of abdominal wall perforated. Johns (1993) suggests that the secondary trocars should be placed medial to the obliterated umbilical arteries and hence through the body of the recti. Garry and Reich (1993) suggest a position lateral to these structures, thus avoiding the recti, and in their technique the venae commitantes are positively identified laparoscopically so that a position lateral to these will be safe.

Superficial epigastric arteries

Transillumination is useful for identifying more superficial vessels such as the superficial epigastrics. Perforation of these tends to cause more superficial hematomata.

Treatment

Prevention of the problem is preferable. However, vascular injuries do occur and may be noted during the procedure as blood dripping down the instrument sheath or, more insidiously, as a developing hematoma. In this situation a number of options are available – simply twisting the sheath through 360° may occlude or tamponade the vessel. Alternatively, a Foley catheter may be inserted through the port, which is then removed, allowing the balloon to be inflated with 10–20 ml of saline. Traction is then applied to the catheter and a small artery forceps is placed across the catheter at the level of the skin to maintain the tamponade.

Bipolar forceps may be passed through another port to diathermy the offending vessel if it can be viewed. If the bleeding point cannot be seen, the vessels immediately adjacent to the site of bleeding may be diathermied and desiccated.

Sutures may also be used – a large curved hand-held needle may be passed through the full thickness of the abdominal wall (inspecting with the laparoscope internally), to occlude the vessels both caudally and cephalad to the bleeding point. A straight needle may be used in the same way, but laparoscopic needle holders will be needed to guide the needle on the peritoneal side under laparoscopic vision. Various equipment companies have developed gadgets for closure of trocar sites and some of these may be used to deal with troublesome bleeding.

Vascular injury may only become apparent postoperatively when the patient presents with symptoms of hypovolemia or with a hematoma. Blood transfusion and laparotomy may then be required. Management of a trocar site hematoma is no different to that for hematomata elsewhere.

TROCAR SITE HERNIAE

There have been a number of reports of herniation of abdominal contents through trocar sites (Liu, 1992; Summitt *et al.*, 1992; Boike *et al.*, 1993; Reich *et al.*, 1993; Ou *et al.*, 1994). Small bowel (or omentum) may be involved, resulting in bowel obstruction and laparotomy. Of the ten reported, seven involved the 12 mm ports that are used with linear stapling devices. These are often placed laterally and if such large ports are used they must be closed in layers. There have recently been reports of herniae with the use of 5 mm ports (Ou *et al.*, 1994), although it is unlikely that bowel would be found in such small hernia sacs.

MAJOR VESSEL INJURY

In the review presented there were two cases of major vessel injury, both involving the Veress needle: in one, the external iliac artery was punctured and the patient underwent immediate laparotomy (and abdominal hysterectomy) and in the other case the infundibulopelvic ligament was injured, presumably causing a vascular injury. In the review this amounts to a risk of 0.06%.

In a review of major vascular injury, Baadsgaard *et al.* (1989) report that the most common occurrence is aortic injury with the Veress needle, at the level of the bifurcation. Injuries to the inferior vena cava, iliac arteries and veins and superior mesenteric vessels have all been reported. Diagnosis is usually immediate and blood will return via the Veress needle and there may be sudden loss of blood pressure. Blood in the peritoneal cavity is rare, so that if the diagnosis is not immediate, a retroperitoneal hematoma will develop resulting in the delayed collapse of the patient, particularly if the vessel is small and the bleeding is venous.

Prevention

Adequate training and good technique are essential. An established safe method of entry into the abdomen is needed along with appreciation of the anatomy; be wary of the thin patient in whom the aorta may lie within 3 cm of the umbilicus and the obese patient in whom anatomical landmarks may be lost. Sharp instruments reduce the force required to pass through the abdominal wall and reduce the risk of overshoot injuries. The temptation to waggle the Veress needle once it is in must be resisted, as this will convert a small puncture into a large tear. A higher pressure pneumoperitoneum (25 mmHg) may be used temporarily so that a large gas pocket is created, into which a short primary trocar is placed. The pressure is then reduced to 15 mmHg for the duration of the procedure (Garry and Reich, 1993).

It is important to appreciate that a retroperitoneal hematoma may be the result of a major vascular injury, which may only slowly expand resulting in postoperative collapse. The surgeon must be aware of this possibility. The CO_2 insufflation pressure may, in some cases, be sufficient to tamponade vessels, so that bleeding only occurs at the completion of the laparoscopy. Hence, it is important to inspect the pelvis at the end of every procedure under low insufflation pressure, less than 8 mmHg.

Treatment

In general, if a major vascular injury is suspected, the Veress needle or trocar should be left in place and a laparotomy performed whilst assistance from a vascular surgeon is sought and the anesthetist resuscitates the patient. Bleeding is stopped with manual compression and the site of the injury identified. The repair may be carried out with simple sutures (Baadsgaard *et al.*, 1989). Similarly, if the diagnosis is delayed and the patient collapses postoperatively, laparotomy, not laparoscopy, is necessary.

BOWEL INJURY

Bowel injury is one of the most serious complications because this diagnosis may be missed at the initial laparoscopy and any delay increases the risk of fecal spillage, peritonitis and death (Garry, 1994). Bowel injury is probably rare but also probably underreported. Querleu *et al.* (1993a), in their large multicenter study, report an incidence of 0.15% for all laparoscopies, which is similar to the rates of 0.06–0.30% reported elsewhere (Levy *et al.*, 1985, 1994; Birns, 1989). The most recent report of the American Association of Gynecologic Laparoscopists (AAGL) (Levy *et al.*, 1994) reports a rate of 0.29% in 80 031 laparoscopies (but the response rate to their questionnaire was only 18%). In the meta-analysis of laparoscopic hysterectomies reported here the rate is 0.32%, which suggests that LH is no more risky than all laparoscopies taken together.

Deaths are known to occur from this complication and have been reported in the newspapers but none are reported in the medical literature. The AAGL has initiated a National Registry of Complications in the USA and the RCOG is currently running a prospective study to assess complications of all types of hysterectomy in the UK.

In Soderstrom's (1993) review of 66 cases of bowel injury during laparoscopy that resulted in litigation, 60 of these cases resulted from trauma that most probably occurred during the initial instrumentation with the Veress needle or the trocar. Several cases occurred despite the use of open laparoscopy (three out of 60) and disposable trocars with safety shields (12 out of 60). This does not necessarily suggest that these measures are not protective because they may have been selectively used in cases where a problem was foreseen. In fact, the AAGL survey reported that the open technique was associated with a 1.2% bowel injury rate and the closed technique with a 0.15% rate – given the very low response rate the only reasonable conclusion is that neither technique is guaranteed safe.

Bowel injury most commonly occurs during the initial insertion of trocars and insufflation needles, but it may also be caused by electrical burns or laceration, as illustrated in Soderstrom's series (1993) and in this meta-analysis. This suggests that hysterectomy *per se* is not the major risk as far as bowel injury is concerned – it is the laparoscopy that is the problem, as there appears to be little difference in the bowel injury rates for hysterectomy alone and all laparoscopic procedures.

In the meta-analysis presented above there were 15 bowel injuries (0.47%), of which there were:

- nine trocar herniae (seven from 12 mm ports);
- three thermal injuries;
- one bowel laceration;
- one internal hernia (loops caught on a loose staple);
- one pelvic abscess (partial colectomy and temporary colostomy).

Treatment of these complications required 11 laparotomies and four laparoscopic repairs. If the nine herniae are excluded, the bowel injury rate is 0.19%, which is lower than that quoted for abdominal hysterectomy.

Death from this complication, although rarely reported in the medical literature, is usually due to delay in diagnosis and treatment (Garry, 1994). Patients who have had any laparoscopic procedure must progressively improve postoperatively and those that do not must be assumed to have a complication until proven otherwise, which may necessitate another laparoscopy (or laparotomy) sooner rather than later. White cell counts, abdominal radiographs or ultrasound may all be normal initially. Observation of a patient who fails to improve is not an option.

Prevention

There will never be a zero rate of complications as long as we continue to push sharp objects into the abdominal cavity. Unfortunately none of the available technological advances has brought about any proven reduction in complication rates. The electrosurgical complications will be dealt with elsewhere (Ch. 11), but will be mentioned briefly here.

Electrical injury may result from unintended damage at the operating site (so-called zone 1) due to surgeon error and heat transfer to adjacent structures, using monopolar or bipolar diathermy. Injuries may also occur outside the operating field within the abdomen (zone 2) as a result of capacitance coupling or insulation failure. Capacitance coupling only occurs when monopolar diathermy is used, but this and insulation failure can both be eliminated when the Electroshield is used.

This device detects any abnormal electrical activity and turns off the current. In addition to this it is important that either all metal or all plastic sheaths are used to prevent injuries around the sheaths that are used (zone 3).

The prevention of traumatic injury to bowel relies on good entry technique and awareness of the potential problems and how to avoid them. The site of insertion of the Veress needle or whether to use the open laparoscopy method described by Hasson is the first decision that has to be made. The most commonly used site is the umbilicus (infra- or intra-umbilical); other sites used are Palmer's point (2–3 cm below the left costal margin in the mid-axillary line at the tip of the ninth rib), suprapubically in the midline, the uterine fundus, the posterior vaginal fornix and the ninth intercostal space in the anterior axillary line. In this department an intraumbilical approach is used, because at this point there is a condensation of fascia and rectus sheath and less fat so that the thickness of the umbilical wall is uniformly thin even in the most obese patients. This is not so with the infraumbilical approach.

In the patient with an old scar close to the umbilicus or with suspected intra-abdominal adhesions, the subcostal approach is preferred because there are rarely adhesions present at this point. Reich uses the ninth intercostal space where he says the peritoneum is more adherent to the underside of the abdominal wall and so prevents 'tenting' of the peritoneum which can lead to misplacement of the tip of the needle. The posterior fornix and the uterine fundus seem particularly hazardous, as bowel may be stuck here as a result of endometriosis which may be unsuspected. The suprapubic site would obviously be a problem in the patient with previous pelvic surgery. These sites have little to offer.

In all cases the Veress needle must be sharp and correctly assembled with an effective spring. The needle should be introduced with the tap open and disconnected from the gas supply. Once the needle is in place, the CO_2 is pumped in at a low flow rate (1 liter per min) and if a good flow is achieved with a low intra-abdominal pressure (less than 5 mmHg), then the needle is correctly placed and the flow may be increased. Other methods of determining correct placement include:

- the 'sniff' test (sniff for bowel gas);
- a drop of saline on the open port of the Veress needle will be sucked in by the slightly negative pressure in the peritoneal cavity;
- injecting 10 ml normal saline (this should be lost and cannot be withdrawn if the needle is in the peritoneal cavity).

A high pressure is then created temporarily (25 mmHg) so that a large pocket of gas overlies the bowel into which a short trocar can be passed. The top of the trocar should be placed in the palm of the hand with the index finger 1 cm behind the tip in order to restrict the depth of travel and the trocar and cannula are then pushed vertically in. All other trocars should be placed under direct vision. If adhesions are suspected and the subcostal approach is used then a 5 mm laparoscope can be used through this port to view the underside of the umbilicus and divide any adhesions that may be present before inserting the 10 mm port and 10 mm laparoscope.

'Open laparoscopy', as described by Hasson, is used in preference by some surgeons; an intra/infraumbilical incision is made and the layers of fat, fascia, sheath and peritoneum are opened in turn using normal laparotomy instruments. A 10/12 mm sheath is then secured using a special port which is sutured into position and the peritoneal cavity is then inflated. An alternative to this is the Visiport (Autosuture, Ascot, UK) which is a trocar with a transparent tip that allows the primary trocar to be inserted with the camera in position behind it, so that the various layers may be visualized as they are traversed. It is not known whether this will prevent bowel injury or just allow the surgeon to identify bowel injury more easily.

Treatment

Veress needle punctures usually do not require repair (Loffer and Pent, 1975). In most cases the patient should be treated with broad-spectrum antibiotics and observed for 24 hours. The patient may then be allowed home with clear instructions to return to hospital if she experiences increasing pain or fever.

Larger lacerations may occur if either the Veress needle is moved around after insertion into the bowel or a trocar or other instrument damages the bowel. The Veress needle should be left in place and a laparotomy performed, with the assistance of a general surgeon if required. In general two layers are advised and as a first layer a purse string may be placed around the needle and tightened as it is withdrawn. Laparoscopic repair with sutures is only advised if the surgeon is extremely experienced. Care must be taken to determine whether the injury is 'through and through' (both sides of the bowel perforated). Colostomy is not indicated for a simple laceration (Soderstrom *et al.*, 1993) and the gynecologist should be present throughout any repair procedure for risk limitation purposes. A smaller laparotomy incision and no colostomy are likely to lead to less medicolegal problems and of course, all patients should be warned of the possibility of a laparotomy. Bowel preparation should be performed if adhesions are suspected or if surgery is required in close proximity to the bowel, such as endometriosis in the rectovaginal septum.

In the situation where the injury is missed at the first operation, then the patient is likely to be ill and may need resuscitation and antibiotic treatment before proceeding to laparotomy. This should be performed by the most experienced general surgeon available with the gynecologist present in theater. The treatment involved will depend upon the injury but may well involve segmental excision of the injured bowel and a temporary defunctioning colostomy.

Electrical injury is rare and will often lead to delayed diagnosis. There may be no perforation initially, just a blanched area, and in these cases 5 cm on either side of the site should be excised to insure that all thermally injured bowel is excised (Soderstrom *et al.*, 1993).

DAMAGE TO OTHER VISCERA

Injury to the stomach is rare (0.027%) (Loffer and Pent, 1975) and is associated with intra-abdominal adhesions and overdistention of the stomach as a result of anesthesia. Some gynecologists advocate the use of an orogastric tube to keep the stomach deflated. These injuries should be managed as for other intestinal injuries. If a Veress needle injury occurs then treatment may be conservative with antibiotics and an orogastric tube (Tripoulos and Griffo, 1993).

Injury to the spleen is also rare and usually occurs during abdominal entry (in the subcostal region), particularly if the spleen is enlarged. The bleeding that occurs with either needle or trocar injury usually subsides and no further treatment is required.

Omental injuries tend to be minor and result in bleeding or emphysema that does not usually require any special treatment. Subcutaneous emphysema is also rarely a problem and tends to subside quickly, particularly with CO_2 as this gas is very soluble. Retroperitoneal insufflation, on the other hand, may be troublesome as it may then prove difficult to penetrate the peritoneum subsequently to allow correct insufflation of the peritoneal cavity (Carter *et al.*, 1993), as well as obscuring anatomical structures.

ANESTHESIA

Carbon dioxide is the most commonly used gas for insufflation of the peritoneal cavity, in part because it is very soluble which reduces the risk of gas embolism which may be fatal (Graff *et al.*, 1959). Absorption may, however, result in a metabolic and respiratory acidosis and this can lead to cardiac arrhythmias (Kokri and Hashim, 1993).

Intra-abdominal pressure may be raised considerably due to the gas insufflation pressure, the Trendelenburg position and the legs being placed in lithotomy. This may make ventilation in obese patients particularly difficult as the diaphragm is splinted, thereby increasing the risk of postoperative atelectasis and pneumonia (Kokri and Hashim, 1993). There is said to be a fall in cardiac output with high insufflation pressures but the significance of this is not known. Pneumothorax, mediastinal emphysema and diaphragmatic rupture may also result from high insufflation and ventilation pressures (Steptoe, 1967).

Vagal stimulation and hemorrhage may lead to hypotension and arrhythmias, which may be exacerbated by CO_2 absorption and the use of halothane (Chantigian and Chantigian, 1993).

There were five transient nerve injuries in this meta-analysis, four involving the sciatic nerve. Both the surgeon and anesthetist must take care with patient positioning, which is crucial for adequate access to the pelvis. Up to 30° of Trendelenburg tilt may be required and the patient's legs must be well supported to allow adequate venous drainage and good access for the surgeon but avoiding any traumatic injury to the patient during these sometimes prolonged procedures.

URETERIC INJURY

In the literature review presented in this chapter the incidence of ureteric injury was at least 0.3% (nine cases in 3189 hysterectomies). At abdominal hysterectomy this rate is quoted as between 0.11% and 0.5% (Amirikia and Evans, 1979; Dicker *et al.*, 1982; Daly and Higgins, 1988). Considering all gynecological surgery, the rates quoted in the literature vary between 0.36% and 2% (Everett and Mattingley, 1956; Mattingley and Borkouf, 1978; Hendry, 1985; Onwudiegwu *et al.*, 1991). This naturally varies with the type of operation being performed

and other contributory factors such as previous surgery, endometriosis, large pelvic masses, adhesions and tumors. Injury to the ureter is said to occur most commonly at the pelvic brim (Daly and Higgins, 1988; Onwudiegwu *et al.*, 1991) and in the ureteric canal (54).

It would appear, then, that LH is not unduly hazardous in this respect. There has been a lot of concern expressed regarding these injuries which have occurred primarily in patients undergoing hysterectomies for so-called benign disease. Certainly some of the reported cases may be directly related to the use of surgical techniques not normally used during abdominal hysterectomy or vaginal hysterectomy, e.g. staples and bipolar diathermy for major vessel hemostasis.

Prevention

Woodland (1992) reported two cases of ureteric injury associated with the use of the endoscopic linear stapler and Nezhat *et al.* (1993) reported three ureteric injuries in two patients associated with the use of the linear stapler. Certainly this device is effective and time saving when used for the ovarian and infundibulopelvic ligaments but its use for securing the uterine arteries has been questioned. Phipps (Phipps *et al.*, 1993) has developed some ureteric stents illuminated by a cold light source which he uses to demonstrate the ureters when securing the uterine arteries. It must be emphasized that these stents cannot be visualized in the ureteric canal immediately adjacent to the uterine artery and, in fact, they must be seen to move even when the stapling clamp has been applied. This should insure safe use of the stapler.

Bipolar diathermy may be used for coaptation and desiccation of the uterine arteries and the ovarian vascular supply. Phipps (1993) has recorded temperatures exceeding 50°C using thermocouples placed adjacent to the ureter when bipolar diathermy is used (50 watts for 8 seconds) and this is sufficient to cause thermal necrosis. However, it is doubtful whether bipolar diathermy needs to be energized for this long in one episode and the fact remains that a large number of laparoscopic hysterectomies are being performed using bipolar diathermy without ureteric problems. It is likely that both bipolar and staples are safe when used with adequate care and skill.

Reich and others have advocated dissecting the ureter out in its pelvic course and using sutures for the major vessels. This technique is surgically sound and requires great skill and time, but it does not guarantee safety. Others have expressed concern about the risk of devascularizing the ureter and, of course, this is not normally required for abdominal hysterectomy for benign disease.

It is impossible to say from the literature review presented whether a subtotal hysterectomy confers any greater safety as regards ureteric injury. It has been estimated that in order to detect a 50% difference risk between two techniques of hysterectomy with respect to any complication that occurs 1% of the time, 4000 cases would be required in each arm of such a study. This is not yet a viable proposition. At this moment in time no ureteric injuries have been reported when using the sub-total approach since only the ascending branches of the uterine artery are occluded.

Diagnosis

In the majority of cases illustrated above the diagnosis is made peroperatively. However, the injury may only present later with anuria (bilateral ureteric injury), a ureterovaginal fistula or urinary ascites (or urinoma). Typically complete ureteric occlusion presents with loin pain and fever between the fourth and ninth postoperative day (Daly and Higgins, 1988). Ultrasound may be used initially for diagnosis, but confirmation of the problem will invariably require IVU. Ideally the diagnosis should be made peroperatively because the injury may then be repaired under the same anesthetic.

There has been one case reported in this literature review of a nephrectomy being performed 15 months after initial surgery, when the patient was found to have an asymptomatic non-functioning kidney. This was an incidental diagnosis and one wonders just how common this might be.

Treatment

This will depend upon the site, size and cause of the injury as well as the timing of presentation. If the injury is recognized immediately at operation a laparotomy is advised. Laparoscopic repair has been carried out (Reich *et al.*, 1993) and a combined cystoscopic and laparoscopic approach has been reported (Neven *et al.*, 1993) using a double-J ureteric catheter inserted cystoscopically and using a laparoscope to guide it between the severed ends of the ureter. In this case a tight fit was obtained and no sutures were required.

At laparotomy, which should be performed by a urologist with the gynecologist in attendance, repair may be carried out by:

- end-to-end anastomosis over a ureteric stent;
- ureteroneocystostomy – particularly if the injury is close to the bladder;
- transuretero-ureterostomy – if a large segment is damaged.

The reader is referred to the text by Hendry (1985).

If diagnosis is delayed, surgical repair is usually delayed until after the insertion of a ureteric stent as a temporary defunctioning procedure. Blandy (Blandy *et al.*, 1991) has suggested that repair should be performed as soon as possible after the diagnosis is made. In his series of 43 patients with ureteral injuries early intervention was possible in the majority and primary healing occurred in all patients.

BLADDER INJURY

This occurred in 1.4% of the laparoscopic hysterectomies reviewed above and this compares with 1.6% after vaginal hysterectomy and 0.3% after abdominal hysterectomy in Dicker's large series (Dicker *et al.*, 1982). The bladder may be injured during insertion of trocars, particularly if it has not been emptied or if it has been pulled cephalad by previous abdominal surgery (e.g. cesarean section). In relation to hysterectomy itself, the bladder may be injured during reflection of the uterovesical fold of the peritoneum and when opening the anterior fornix of the vagina (whether laparoscopically or vaginally) and when closing the vault after the hysterectomy is completed. Injuries may occur as a direct result of trauma with scissors, graspers, pushers, the laser, electrosurgical instruments and sutures. Care must be taken at all times, particularly when there has been previous surgery or endometriosis affecting the uterovesical pouch. Injury may be delayed if it is due to thermal necrosis or to an expanding hematoma.

Diagnosis

This may be immediate or delayed until the postoperative period. Bladder lacerations will leak urine into the peritoneal cavity, the perivesical tissues and the cave of Retzius if the peritoneum is intact (extraperitoneal) and the vagina. If the diagnosis is not immediate then the patient will present later, usually with suprapubic pain, possibly fever or a leak of urine or suprapubic fullness. Sudden hematuria due to a hematoma discharging may also be an indication of bladder trauma. There may be peritoneal signs of ascites and diagnosis is usually made by cystoscopy, retrograde cystography and possibly abdominal ultrasound.

Prevention

The bladder must be emptied and preferably kept empty. Some surgeons favor leaving a Foley catheter *in situ* for the duration of all hysterectomies rather than just drainage at the start of the procedure. Clearly care must be taken in the presence of previous surgery, endometriosis and pelvic inflammatory disease. Awareness of the possibility of bladder trauma must always be high in these cases and, if necessary, methylene blue may be instilled into the bladder during the procedure or 5 ml of indigo carmine may be injected intravenously. Some surgeons are now performing cystoscopy at the end of laparoscopic hysterectomies both to view the ureteric orifices and confirm there is urine flow into the bladder and also to inspect the bladder cavity itself.

Care with the use of electrosurgical and laser energy near to the bladder is always required. Thermal necrosis may present later with a vesicovaginal fistula and the area of trauma may be large. Hemostasis must be sound, as again an enlarging hematoma may cause pressure necrosis of a relatively large area. Sutures must always be placed with care, particularly along the vaginal vault, either laparoscopically or vaginally as quite a number of the urinary tract injuries described in the review above were caused at this stage.

Treatment

Immediate

If the diagnosis is made immediately, then repair should be carried out immediately. Laparoscopic repair has been reported (Reich and McGlynn, 1990) but should only be performed by very experienced laparoscopic surgeons. A laparotomy will be required unless the laceration can be reached vaginally. Avoidance of a laparotomy incision will reduce the chances of subsequent litigation, but the surgeon's priority must be a good repair. Repairs are generally carried out in two layers traditionally with chromic catgut sutures (Corrier and Sandler, 1986), although Vicryl and PDS have been used (Reich and McGlynn, 1990). A purse string may be used around a trocar injury and the repair completed in 2–3 layers if necessary (Bassil *et al.*, 1993). Some authors advise interrupted sutures at all levels

(Lawson, 1972) while others prefer running locking sutures for water-tightness in the mucosa and muscularis and interrupted to the adventitial layer (Corrier and Sandler, 1986).

In all cases the bladder must be drained for 7–10 days postoperatively with either a suprapubic or urethral catheter. Suprapubic catheters should be placed away from the site of the laceration. Sterile urine is necessary for adequate healing and microscopy must be carried out frequently before, during and after treatment along with appropriate antibiotic cover.

Delayed

Presentation occurs with a vesicovaginal fistula or intraperitoneal or other extraperitoneal leak. In this situation consultation with urological experts is advised. Small leaks may resolve and a trial of conservative treatment, i.e. catheter on continuous drainage with antibiotic cover, is worth considering because small defects often close (Hendry, 1985). Extraperitoneal leaks may often be managed with a large or Foley catheter as the bladder will often heal and the extravasated urine will be reabsorbed.

Other bladder problems

Urinary tract infection occurred in 0.8% of cases in the review above and this compares with 3.4% following vaginal hysterectomy and 7% following abdominal hysterectomy in Dicker's series (Dicker *et al.*, 1982). Certainly this problem appears much less frequent following LH but this may simply be a failure to report it as patients spend the majority of their convalescence at home following a LH. It is also possible that there may be technical benefits in the way the bladder is dissected at LH.

Urine retention appears to be infrequent following LH and this may be related to the degree of postoperative pain that patients experience. This is certainly much reduced following LH compared with abdominal hysterectomy (Phipps *et al.*, 1993).

FEBRILE MORBIDITY

Dicker *et al.* (1982) report the incidence of febrile morbidity to be 32.3% after abdominal hysterectomy and 15.3% after vaginal hysterectomy. In the literature review presented here the incidence is 4.3%. This includes urinary tract infection, pneumonia, pelvic infection, trocar cellulitis and infection. Apart from the obvious benefits to the patient, this may produce quite a saving in health authority budgets in relation to antibiotic drug costs and postoperative stay in hospital. However, there may be a significant methodological problem in that patients discharged home early after LH may not have frequent monitoring of their temperatures and so febrile morbidity may simply be missed. Additionally, prophylactic antibiotics are always administered at the time of LH.

VAGINAL VAULT PROBLEMS

Vault hematoma, cellulitis and pelvic abscess/ hematoma may occur with all types of hysterectomy. The incidence appears to be slightly lower with laparoscopic assisted vaginal hysterectomy (1%) compared to 3.3% in vaginal hysterectomy and 4.4% in abdominal hysterectomy (Dicker *et al.*, 1982). This may certainly reflect the fact that hemostasis is checked at the end of the laparoscopic procedure and even very small bleeding points may be cauterized with great accuracy. It is important to carry out this final inspection at low intraabdominal pressure so that small vessel bleeding is not tamponaded by the high pressure pneumoperitoneum.

Following subtotal hysterectomy persistent menstruation occurs infrequently, as does mucorrhea. It does, however, give rise to some women requesting removal of the cervical stump which is sometimes a technically difficult operation. Unfortunately, there have been insufficient numbers performed to make any valid statistical comparison.

LAPAROTOMY

In the review presented above there is a surprisingly high number of laparotomies (3.5%). This includes laparotomy done for conversion to abdominal hysterectomy for whatever reason, as well as management of complications either at the time of initial surgery or at a later laparotomy and so this figure represents the overall risk of a patient experiencing a laparotomy (included in this figure are all the laparotomies performed for postoperative herniae). It compares well with Dicker's study which showed a 5.1% risk of unintended major surgery after vaginal hysterectomy and 1.7% after abdominal hysterectomy. It may be possible that, as the surgeon's experience increases, fewer laparotomies are performed. There is some evidence that this is not the case, as surgeons may take on more complex laparoscopic cases as their expertise increases and this may negate the learning curve effect (Ou *et al.*, 1994).

PULMONARY EMBOLUS

Following abdominal hysterectomy the pulmonary embolus rate is 0.2% and following vaginal hysterectomy, it is zero in Dicker's study. The rate quoted in the literature review here is comparable. Certainly the same precautions against deep vein thrombosis should be taken with LH as are taken with abdominal hysterectomy.

TOTAL OR SUBTOTAL?

On the basis of the current literature there is no evidence to suggest that subtotal LH is any safer than total LH. This may simply be a problem of numbers as there are no large series of subtotal hysterectomies. It is claimed that complications with the vaginal cuff are reduced as there is no vaginal cuff and because the vaginal vault is not opened, there is less risk of pelvic and vault sepsis. Complications arising from dissection of the bladder may be reduced as less mobilization is required and ureteric injuries may also be reduced as the vaginal vault is not closed at subtotal hysterectomy, although the uterine arteries still have to be divided, albeit only the ascending branches.

There has been a great deal of debate concerning sexual function after hysterectomy. It may improve (Virtanen *et al.*, 1993; Carlson *et al.*, 1994) or deteriorate – the reports are confusing. The much-quoted study by Kilkku *et al.* (1993), comparing total abdominal and subtotal abdominal hysterectomy, was not randomized and showed no definite statistically significant difference in outcome (libido and orgasm frequency) between the two groups. There was a statistically significant reduction in orgasm frequency after hysterectomy but not after subtotal hysterectomy, whereas when the two groups were compared pre- and then postoperatively there was no significant difference – that is statistical confusion! In both groups there was an increase in the number of women with weak or absent libido after hysterectomy. If there is any significant difference between the two groups and this is felt to be important, then logically vaginal hysterectomy could become obsolete.

LONG-TERM MORBIDITY

Long-term changes in bladder function following traditional abdominal and vaginal hysterectomy have been reported as well as psychiatric morbidity, fatigue, sexual dysfunction and bowel dysfunction (Virtanen *et al.*, 1993; Carlson *et al.*, 1994). Some of these effects are beneficial and some are detrimental. There are no data to suggest that the laparoscopic approach fares any better or worse than the conventional approaches, although with the passage of time, differences may become apparent.

REFERENCES

Amirikia, H. and Evans, T.N. (1979) Ten-year review of hysterectomies: trends, indications, and risks. *Am J Obstet Gynecol*, **134**, 431–7.

Arbogast, J.D., Welch, R.A., Riza, E.D. *et al.* (1994) Laparoscopically assisted vaginal hysterectomy appears to be an alternative to total abdominal hysterectomy. *J Laparoendosc Surg*, **4**, 185–90.

Baadsgaard, S.E., Bille, S. and Egeblad, K. (1989) Major vascular injury during gynecologic laparoscopy. *Acta Obstet Gynecol Scand*, **68**, 283–5.

Bassil, S., Nisolle, M. and Donnez, J. (1993) Complications of endoscopic surgery in gynaecology. *Gynecol Endosc*, **2**, 199–209.

Birns, M.T. (1989) Inadvertent instrumental perforation of the colon during laparoscopy: nonsurgical repair. *Gastrointest Endosc*, **35**, 54–6.

Blandy, J.P., Badenoch, D.F., Fowler, G.G. *et al.* (1991) Early repair of iatrogenic injury to the ureter or bladder after gynaecological surgery. *J Urol*, **146**, 761–5.

Boike, G.M., Elfstrand, E.P., DelPriore, G. *et al.* (1993) Laparoscopically assisted vaginal hysterectomy in a university hospital: report of 82 cases and comparison with abdominal and vaginal hysterectomy. *Am J Obstet Gynecol*, **168**, 1690–701.

Bronitsky, C., Payne, R.J., Stuckey, S. and Wilkins, D. (1993) A comparison of laparoscopically assisted vaginal hysterectomy vs traditional total abdominal and vaginal hysterectomies. *J Gynecol Surg*, **9**, 219–25.

Bruhat, M.A., Wattiez, A., Mage, G. *et al.* (1994) Hysterectomie percoelioscopique. *Ref Gynecol Obstet*, **2**, 53–67.

Carlson, K.J., Miller, B.A. and Fowler, F.J. Jr (1994) The Maine women's health study. I. Outcomes of hysterectomy. *Obstet Gynecol*, **83**, 556–65.

Carter, J., Fowler, J., Carson, L. and Twiggs, L.B. (1993) Management of complications of laparoscopic surgery in gynaecology. *Gynecol Endosc*, **2**, 175–80.

Casey, M.J., Garcia-Padial, J., Johnson, C. *et al.* (1994) A critical analysis of laparoscopic assisted vaginal hysterectomies compared with vaginal hysterectomies unassisted by laparoscopy and transabdominal hysterectomies. *J Gynecol Surg*, **10**, 7–14.

Chantigian, R.C. and Chantigian, P.D.M. (1993) Anaesthesia for laparoscopy, in *Complications of Laparoscopy and Hysteroscopy*, (eds R.S. Corfman, M.P. Diamond and A. DeCherney), Blackwell Scientific, Boston, pp. 11–21.

Corrier, J.N. and Sandler, C.M. (1986) Management of the ruptured bladder: 7 years experience with 111 cases. *J Trauma*, **26**, 830–3.

Daly, J.W. and Higgins, K.A. (1988) Injury to the ureter during gynecologic surgical procedures. *Surg Gynecol Obstet*, **168**, 19–22.

Dicker, R.C., Greenspan, J.R., Strauss, L.T. *et al.* (1982) Complications of abdominal and vaginal hysterectomy among women of reproductive age in the United States. *Am J Obstet Gynecol*, **144**, 841–7.

Donnez, J. and Nisolle, M. (1993) Laparoscopic supracervical (subtotal) hysterectomy (LASH). *J Gynecol Surg*, **9**, 91–4.

Everett, H.S. and Mattingley, R.F. (1956) Urinary tract injuries resulting from pelvic surgery. *Am J Obstet Gynecol*, **71**, 502.

Ewen, S.P. and Sutton, C.J.G. (1994) Initial experience with supracervical hysterectomy and removal of the cervical tranaformation zone. *Br J Obstet Gynaecol*, **101**, 225–8.

Garcia-Padial, J., Sotolongo, J., Casey, M.J. *et al.* (1992) Laparoscopy-assisted vaginal hysterectomy: report of 75 consecutive cases. *J Gynecol Surg*, **8**, 81–5.

Garry, R. (1994) The Achilles heel of minimal access surgery. *Gynecol Endosc*, **3**, 201–2.

Garry, R. and Hercz, P. (1995) Initial experience with laparoscopic assisted Doderlein hysterectomy – an improved method for laparoscopic hysterectomy. *Br J Obstet Gynaecol*, **102**, 307–10.

Garry, R. and Reich, H. (1993) Basic techniques for advanced laparoscopic surgery, in *Laparoscopic Hysterectomy*, (eds. R. Garry and H. Reich), Blackwell Scientific, Oxford, pp. 46–78.

Graff, T.D., Arbogast, N.R., Phillips, O.C. *et al.* (1959) Gas embolism. A comparative study of air and CO_2 as embolic agents in the systemic venous system. *Am J Obstet Gynecol*, **78**, 249–65.

Grainger, D.A., Bowen, L., Delmere, J.E. *et al.* (1992) Laparoscopic assisted vaginal hysterectomy: 50 consecutive cases compared to the traditional vaginal approach. *Fertil Steril* (Annual Meeting Program Supplement), 25–6.

Hasson, H.M., Rotman, C., Rana, N. *et al.* (1993) Experience with laparoscopic hysterectomy. *J Am Assoc Gynecol Laparosc*, **1**, 1–11.

Hendry, W.F. (1988) Urinary tract injuries during gynaecological surgery, in *Progress in Obstetrics and Gynaecology*, (ed. J.W.W. Studd), Churchill Livingstone, Edinburgh, pp. 362–77.

Houreabie, J.A. and Bruhat, M.A. (1993) Laparoscopic hysterectomy using endo-GIA staples and a device for presenting the vaginal fornices. *J Gynecol Endosc*, **2**, 65–72.

Howard, F.M. and Sanchez, R. (1993) A comparison of laparoscopically assisted vaginal hysterectomy and abdominal hysterectomy. *J Gynecol Surg*, **9**, 83–90.

Hunter, R.W. and McCartney, A.J. (1993) Can laparoscopic assisted hysterectomy safely replace abdominal hysterectomy? *Br J Obstet Gynaecol*, **100**, 932–4.

Johns, D.A. (1993) Perforation of the inferior epigastric vessels, in *Complications of Laparoscopy and Hysteroscopy*, (eds. R.S. Corfman, M.P. Diamond and A.H. DeCherney), Blackwell Scientific, Boston, pp. 38–41.

Jones, R.A. (1995) Complications of laparoscopic hysterectomy – 250 cases. *Gynecol Endosc*, **4**, 95–9.

Kilkku, P., Gronroos, M., Hirvonen, T. and Rauramo, L. (1983) Supravaginal uterine amputation vs. hysterectomy. Effects on libido and orgasm. *Acta Obstet Gynecol Scand*, **62**, 147–52.

Kokri, M.S. and Hashim, F. (1993) Anaesthesia for gynaecological endoscopic surgery, in *Laparoscopic Hysterectomy*, (eds R. Garry and H. Reich), Blackwell Scientific, Oxford, pp. 167–70.

Lawson, K.J. (1972) Vesical fistulae into the vaginal vault. *Br J Urol*, **72**, 868–72.

Levy, B.S., Soderstrom, R.M. and Dail, D.H. (1985) Bowel injuries during laparoscopy: gross anatomy and histology. *J Reprod Med*, **30**, 168–72.

Levy, B.S., Hulka, J.F., Peterson, H.B. and Phillips, J.M. (1994) Operative laparoscopy: American Association of Gynecologic Laparoscopists 1993 membership survey. *J Am Assoc Gynecol Laparosc*, **1**, 301–5.

Liu, C.Y. (1992) Laparoscopic hysterectomy: report of 215 cases. *Gynecol Endosc*, **1**, 73–7.

Liu, C.Y. (1993a) Laparoscopic hysterectomy. *Gynecol Endosc*, **2**, 73–5.

Liu, C.Y. (1993b) Complications of laparoscopic hysterectomy: prevention, recognition and management, in *Complications of Laparoscopy and Hysteroscopy*, (eds. R.S. Corfman, M.P. Diamond and A. DeCherney), Blackwell Scientific, Boston, pp. 160–6.

Loffer, F. and Pent, D. (1975) Indications, contra-indications and complications of laparoscopy. *Obstet Gynecol Surv*, **30**, 407–27.

Mattingley, R.F. and Borkouf, H.I. (1978) Acute operative injury to the lower urinary tract. *Clin Obstet Gynecol*, **5**, 123.

Mencaglia, L., van Herendael, B., Tantini, C. and Stampini, A. (1994) Laparoscopic assisted vaginal hysterectomy: evaluation of benefits of laparoscopic hysterectomy. *Gynecol Endosc*, **3**, 209–11.

Neven, P., Vandeursen, H., Baert, L. and Koninckx, P.R. (1993) Ureteric injury at laparoscopic surgery: the endoscopic management. *Gynecol Endosc*, **2**, 45–6.

Nezhat, C., Nezhat, F., Bess, O. *et al.* (1993) Injuries associated with the use of a linear stapling device during operative laparoscopy: review of diagnosis, management, and prevention. *J Gynecol Surg*, **9**, 145–50.

Nezhat, F., Nezhat, C., Gordon, S. and Wilkin, C.S.T. (1992) Laparoscopic versus abdominal hysterectomy. *J Reprod Med*, **37**, 247–50.

O'Connor, D., Molloy, D. and Guest, A. Complications of 216 laparoscopic assisted vaginal hysterectomies. Personal communication.

Onwudiegwu, U., Makinde, O.O., Badejo, O.A. *et al.* (1991) Ureteric injuries associated with gynecologic surgery. *Int J Gynecol Obstet*, **34**, 235–8.

Ou, C.S., Beadle, E., Presthus, J. and Smith, M. (1994) A multicenter review of 839 laparoscopic assisted vaginal hysterectomies. *J Am Assoc Gynecol Laparosc*, **1**, 417–22.

Phipps, J.H. (1993) Thermometry studies with bipolar diathermy during hysterectomy. *Gynecol Endosc*, **3**, 5–7.

Phipps, J.H., John, M., Hassanaien, M. and Saeed, M. (1993) Laparoscopic and laparoscopically assisted vaginal hysterectomy: a series of 114 cases. *Gynecol Endosc*, **2**, 7–12.

Querleu, D., Chevallier, L., Chapron, C. and Bruhat, M.A. (1993a) Complications of gynaecological laparoscopic surgery. A French multicentre collaborative study. *Gynecol Endosc*, **2**, 3–6.

Querleu, D., Cosson, M., Parmentier, D. and Debodinance, P. (1993b) The impact of laparoscopic surgery on vaginal hysterectomy. *Gynecol Endosc*, **2**, 89–91.

Reich, H. and McGlynn, F. (1990) Laparoscopic repair of bladder injury. *Obstet Gynecol*, **76**, 909–10.

Reich, H., McGlynn, F. and Sekel, L. (1993) Total laparoscopic hysterectomy. *Gynecol Endosc*, **2**, 59–63.

Saye, W.B., Espy, G.B., Bishop, M.R. *et al.* (1993) Laparoscopic assisted Doderlein hysterectomy: a rational alternative to traditional abdominal hysterectomy. *Surg Laparosc Endosc*, **3**, 88–94.

Schwartz, R.O. (1993) Complications of laparoscopic hysterectomy. *Obstet Gynecol*, **81**, 1022–4.

Soderstrom, R.M. (1993) Bowel injury litigation after laparoscopy. *J Am Assoc Gynecol Laparosc*, **1**, 74–7.

Soderstrom, R.M., Levinson, C. and Levy, B.S. (1993) Complications of operative laparoscopy, in *Operative Laparoscopy – The Masters' Technique*, (ed. R.M. Soderstrom), Raven Press, New York, pp. 187–97.

Steptoe, P.C. (1967) *Laparoscopy in Gynaecology*, ES. Livingstone, Edinburgh, pp. 30–4.

Summitt, R.L. Jr, Stovall, T.G., Lipscomb, G.H. *et al.* (1992) Randomised comparison of laparoscopy-assisted vaginal hysterectomy with standard vaginal hysterectomy in an outpatient setting. *Obstet Gynecol*, **80**, 895–901.

Tripoulos, J. and Grifo, J. (1993) Trocar injuries to the stomach, in *Complications of Laparoscopy and Hysteroscopy*, (eds. R.S. Corfman, M.P. Diamond and A. DeCherney), Blackwell Scientific, Boston, pp. 60–3.

Viranen, H., Makinen, J., Tenho, T. *et al.* (1993) Effects of abdominal hysterectomy on urinary and sexual symptoms. *Br J Urol*, **72**, 868–72.

Wood, C., Maher, P. and Hill, D. (1994a) Current status of laparoscopic associated hysterectomy. *Gynecol Endosc*, **3**, 75–84.

Wood, C., Maher, P., Hill, D. and Lolatgis, N. (1994b) Laparovaginal hysterectomy. *Aust NZ J Obstet Gynaecol*, **34**, 81–4.

Woodland, M.B. (1992) Ureter injury during laparoscopy-assisted vaginal hysterectomy with the endoscopic linear stapler. *Am J Obstet Gynecol*, **167**, 756–7.

A. Pooley

INTRODUCTION

Uterine leiomyomata are the commonest solid tumors of the female genital tract and will be found in 20–25% of women aged over 35 years (Smith, 1952). However, only 20–50% of women with fibroids will have symptoms referrable to them, the common complaints being menstrual disorders, pressure symptoms and the appreciation of an abdominopelvic mass (Buttram and Reiter, 1981). In the absence of effective long-term medical therapy traditional treatment has involved major surgery. Before the advent of endoscopic alternatives, uterine fibroids were the main indication for up to 25% of the 600 000 hysterectomies performed annually in the United States, with a further 18 000 abdominal myomectomies per year performed to preserve fertility potential (NCHS, 1987).

Interest and enthusiasm for endoscopic alternatives to traditional gynecological surgery has grown exponentially in the last ten years, initially amongst gynecologists themselves but soon followed by health care providers and the female public at large. An increasing number of women seek 'organ-preserving' surgery and request myomectomy rather than hysterectomy and other minimal access treatments for the various problems fibroids may cause.

When discussing endoscopic therapy for fibroids it is convenient to deal with hysteroscopic and laparoscopic approaches separately, but they are not mutually exclusive and will be complementary in virtually all cases.

HYSTEROSCOPIC SURGERY

Submucous and intramural fibroids may cause menstrual disorders and anemia, dysmenorrhea, infertility, early pregnancy loss and complications in later pregnancy (Buttram and Reiter, 1981). Often missed and rarely helped by blind curretage (Wamsteker, 1984), fibroids impinging on the endometrial cavity can be clearly seen with modern diagnostic hysteroscopy. In 1976 Neuwirth and Amin described excision of submucous fibroids using semirigid scissors, moving on to use electrosurgical resection two years later (Neuwirth, 1978). Two modalities are now in common use, with many proponents of both electrosurgery and the use of the Nd-YAG laser.

A classification of submucous fibroids introduced by Wamsteker and adopted by the European Society of Hysteroscopy in 1990 is now in common use (Figure 5.1). This describes fibroids as grade 0 when pedunculate and entirely within the uterine cavity, grade I when less than 50% of the fibroid is beneath the level of the endometrium and grade II when the majority of the fibroid is intramural.

Gynecological Endoscopic Surgery. Edited by C.J.G. Sutton. Published in 1997 by Chapman & Hall, London.
ISBN 0 412 58040 3.

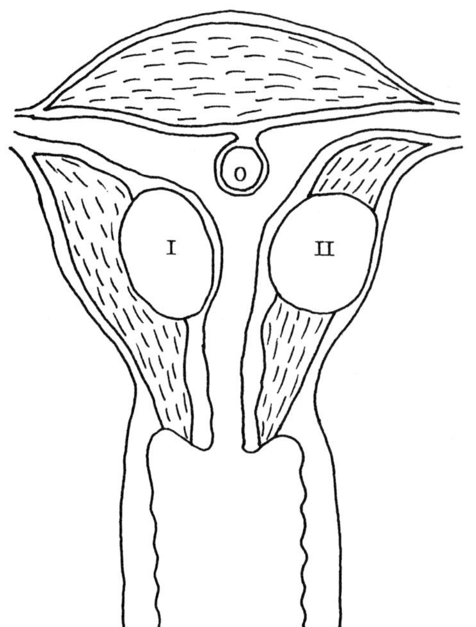

Figure 5.1 Classification of submucous fibroids, grades 0, I and II.

PREOPERATIVE PREPARATION

The high quality images from modern transvaginal ultrasonography are of great value preoperatively and may be enhanced by placing a small amount of 0.9% saline solution into the uterine cavity (saline infusion sono-hysterography). A detailed three-dimensional map of the uterus will allow greater confidence when dealing with intramural fibroids and will detect deeper fibroids, given that there are frequently multiple fibroids present. Preoperative treatment with gonadotropin hormone-releasing hormone (GnRH) analogs is used by many practitioners. Having been shown to shrink fibroids and correct associated anemia (Filicori *et al.*, 1983), it is disappointing that the effects wear off after stopping the therapy, with the return of both the fibroid volume and the symptoms (Matta *et al.*, 1988). Reduction in volume of up to 38% is common but variable, with a lesser effect on smaller grade 0 fibroids (Donnez *et al.*, 1989).

The use of GnRH analogs will render the endometrium atrophic and reduce the volume of tissue needing to be removed. This will improve vision, making the procedure easier and quicker, and reduce fluid absorption. Prolonged use, however, may induce a fibrous reaction, making surgery more difficult (Hamou, 1993).

UTERINE DISTENTION

Hysteroscopic surgery is always performed using a distention medium, the commonest being 1.5% glycine, a smaller number using 4% sorbitol. For Nd-YAG laser surgery there are proponents for both fluid and carbon dioxide distention. Using carbon dioxide, the Nd-YAG energy needed is approximately half that required for fluid distention.

One must always be alert to the dangers of air or gas embolism. Air embolism can occur whenever an open vein is exposed to air at greater pressure than the venous pressure. This can occur if air is allowed to enter the uterine cavity when the patient is positioned with a Trendelenburg tilt, especially if the patient is breathing spontaneously. Carbon dioxide uterine distention should only be performed using a device specifically designed for that purpose incorporating both pressure and flow control mechanisms. The dangers of using sapphire-tipped laser fibers with the so-called coaxial gas cooling system are now fully realized, with cases of severe brain damage and death recorded (Baggish and Daniell, 1989).

OPERATIVE TECHNIQUES

The procedure performed will depend on the site and size of the fibroids, the symptoms caused and the wishes of the woman.

Grade 0 fibroids of less than 5 cm diameter are relatively easy to deal with. The pedicle can be divided by electroresection, the YAG laser fiber or a polyp snare (McLucas, 1992). Vaporization is also possible using a grooved rollerbarrel recently described by Brookes (1996). This device, borrowed from the urologists, utilizes the electrosurgical principle of 'edge density' to vaporize fibroids at 200 watts. The author acknowledges the higher risk of perforation at such power settings. The detached fibroid can be fragmented and removed or left in the cavity to autolyze or be expelled during the first menses after the procedure (Donnez, 1993).

For grade II fibroids a two-stage procedure is often adopted. This is based on the finding that the deeper intramural portion, if left behind, will be found to protrude into the cavity at a second visit after two months of GnRH analog therapy, facilitating complete removal. Endometrial resection or ablation can be performed at the same time for women with menstrual disorders whose family is complete. The greater confidence afforded by laparoscopic supervision of such procedures during concomitant sterilization suggests that one should make use of this facility for deeper seated fibroids.

RESULTS

The removal of submucous fibroids will often correct excessive menstrual loss. An objective reduction in flow of 77% has been demonstrated by the resection of a single 1 cm fibroid (Broadbent and Magos, 1995). Up to 90% of women will have excessive menstrual loss controlled (Wamsteker, 1993), but failure rates of 22% are described when combined with endometrial ablation for multiple fibroids, when recurrence is more likely (Donnez, 1993). For women whose only identifiable infertility factor is submucous fibroids conception rates of 66% have been described for both electroresection (Hamou, 1993) and Nd-YAG laser surgery (Donnez, 1993).

LAPAROSCOPIC MYOMECTOMY

Traditionally open myomectomy has been performed for women with fibroids causing infertility or pressure effects who contemplate further pregnancy. Laparoscopic myomectomy is indicated for the same conditions, but is also used for women who wish to have alleviation of their symptoms of abnormal bleeding and pressure without the need to lose their uterus. The laparoscopic removal of asymptomatic fibroids is of dubious value, even if pedunculate and requiring little surgical effort. That myomectomy can be performed laparoscopically has been known for some time (Semm and Metler, 1980), but even with enormous advances in instrument technology and surgical experience, this procedure has yet to be widely adopted.

PREOPERATIVE PREPARATION

Preoperative ultrasonography is of great value, as some intramural fibroids palpable at open myomectomy may be missed at laparoscopy. The majority of proponents of this procedure choose the benefits of preoperative GnRH analogs, accepting the possible increased difficulty in enucleating the fibroids. As with any surgical procedure, a detailed description should be given to the patient beforehand, including likely outcomes and possible complications. For laparoscopic myomectomy this should include the risk of needing to proceed to a laparotomy and even to hysterectomy.

OPERATIVE TECHNIQUES

The techniques used for advanced laparoscopic surgery embrace the principles of surgery for infertility, those of magnification, minimal tissue handling and trauma, scrupulous hemostasis and the avoidance of desiccation. As with open myomectomy, at laparoscopy the uterine serosa is incised, the fibroid is dissected free and the defect in the myometrium and serosa is repaired. There is the added problem of retrieving the fibroid from the peritoneal cavity. Hemostasis can be a problem, with some authors using a vasoconstrictor as a chemical tourniquet. Dubuisson and his colleagues in France are not permitted to use this technique and find preoperative use of GnRH analogs sufficient.

The uterine incision is effected with cutting monopolar diathermy or lasers, with proponents of both carbon dioxide and Nd-YAG modalities. Dubuisson uses large forceps, a monopolar hook and curved scissors to enucleate the fibroid (Dubuisson and Chapron, 1995). Others use a combination of laparoscopic myomectomy screws, aquadissection and lasers (Daniell and Gurley, 1991; Nezhat *et al.*, 1991). The endometrial cavity is not intentionally opened and some use methylene blue to stain the endometrium to help identify inadvertent breach of the cavity. The myometrial defect is closed using sutures, the concern being to avoid a weakness which could rupture during subsequent pregnancy. Historically open myomectomy has a low risk of subsequent uterine rupture (Davids, 1952) and there are two case reports of rupture at 34 weeks amenorrhea after laparoscopic myomectomy (Harris, 1992; Dubuisson *et al.*, 1995).

Small fibroids less than 2 cm in diameter can usually be removed easily through the abdominal portals. Larger fibroids can be extracted intact via an enlarged portal or posterior colpotomy or morcellated. Various morcellation techniques are described ranging from the insertion of a small scalpel through the abdominal wall (the poor man's morcellator) to specific electromechanical devices.

One of the main drawbacks of laparoscopic myomectomy is the time the procedure takes. The average time described in the literature is in the order of two hours (Nezhat *et al.*, 1991; Dubuisson *et al.*, 1995), with cases lasting seven hours being recorded (Hasson *et al.*, 1992). This led Dubuisson to set upper limits of up to four fibroids no more than 8–10 cm in diameter. Nezhat has described the technique of laparoscopic assisted myomectomy (Nezhat *et al.*, 1994). Under laparoscopic control the uterus is brought up to a minilaparotomy incision, making the operation easier and quicker

and possibly allowing more secure closure of the intramural defect.

COMPLICATIONS AND RESULTS

Adhesion formation has long been known to result from open myomectomy, with more adhesions occurring on posterior uterine incisions (Tulandi *et al.*, 1993). GoreTex (polytetrafluoroethylene) has been shown to reduce adhesions at open myomectomy (Myomectomy Adhesion Multicenter Study Group, 1995), but dense adhesions have been recorded despite its use at laparoscopic myomectomy (Daniell and Gurley, 1991). Adhesions will probably occur in up to two-thirds of cases, with fewer adhesions if the serosa is not repaired with sutures. There is little information on the impact of these adhesions, but some advocate an early second-look laparoscopy to break down any that have formed (Hasson *et al.*, 1992). Pregnancy rates of up to 70% are recorded after laparoscopic myomectomy (Hasson *et al.*, 1992), but most of the literature focuses on surgical technique rather than long-term outcomes. There is a 5–30% recurrence rate after open myomectomy, with 20–25% of women requiring further surgery, usually hysterectomy (Candiani *et al.*, 1991). One must assume similar figures will result after the laparoscopic approach.

MYOLYSIS

Laparoscopic myomectomy requires considerable surgical skill and theater time. As an alternative therapy laparoscopic coagulation of fibroids has been developed. The intention is to devascularize the tumor, leading to ischemic aseptic necrobiosis and involution without hemorrhagic infarction. Initially used via the hysteroscope, the thermal effect of the Nd-YAG laser can be used laparoscopically (Manhes and Lesec, 1988). While some use a bare laser fiber (Nisolle *et al.*, 1993), others use a fluid-cooled needle to insert the laser fiber into subserosal and intramural fibroids

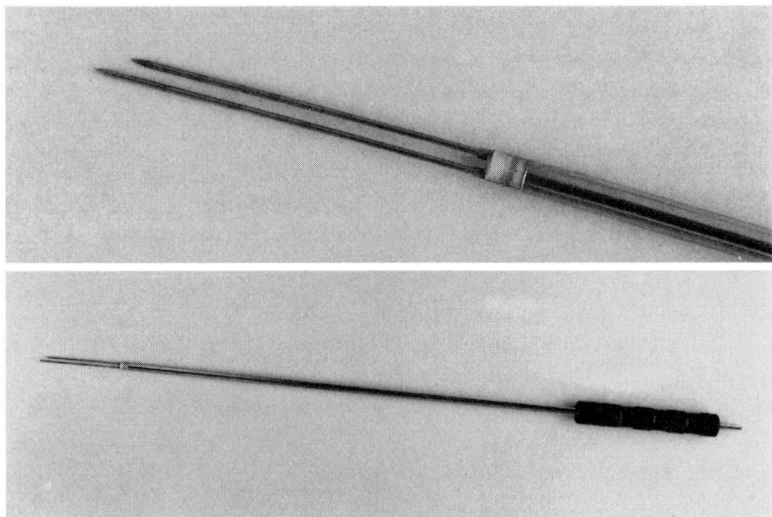

Figure 5.2 Bipolar myolysis probe with proximal insulation.

(Gallinat, 1995). Gallinat went on to develop a bipolar needle probe to cause electrocoagulation within the fibroid (Gallinat, 1995) (Plate 1). Both techniques require multiple insertions 5–10 mm apart to 'pepper' the fibroids, causing zones of coagulation. Typically 20–80 watts of Nd-YAG energy are used, with 70–120 watts using the bipolar probe.

Ultrasonography is required to accurately localize the intramural extent of the fibroids and hysteroscopic surgery is used to deal with submucous fibroids and to perform endometrial ablation at the same time if indicated. The procedure is confined to women no longer wishing to preserve their fertility due to concerns regarding asymptomatic cyst formation with weakening of the uterine wall. Fibroid volume reductions of 60–70% are reported, which is similar to the effect of GnRH analogs, but appear to be permanent (Goldfarb, 1992; Nisoue *et al.*, 1993; Gallinat, 1995).

Philips (1995) has reported a series of 97 women with symptomatic fibroids treated with myolysis using the bipolar probe, the Nd-YAG laser or a combination of the two. In 39 of these women a concomitant transcervical resection of the endometrium was performed, 19 of whom also had resection of the submucous portion of one or more fibroids. The procedure was restricted to cases who showed a greater than 25% reduction in total uterine volume after three months of GnRH analog therapy. Using transvaginal ultrasonography preoperatively and at six and 12 months after surgery, an 81% reduction in total uterine volume was demonstrated, with an 87% reduction in total fibroid volume. One concern is that severe pain might result from acute hemorrhagic degeneration. In Philips' series of 97 cases this occurred only once, in the one woman who declined to have the GnRH analog pretreatment for three months.

As with laparoscopic myomectomy, there is concern regarding adhesion formation. In the series reported by Nisolle *et al.* (1993) dense fibrous adhesions to the small bowel were seen in all of seven cases who had a second-look laparoscopy six months after Nd-YAG laser myolysis. Philips has also found adhesions after using Nd-YAG myolysis, but none in 13 women who had bipolar coagulation using an insulated probe which avoids significant coagulation of the serosa (JEMD Medical, Hicksville, USA) (Figure 5.2). A further con-

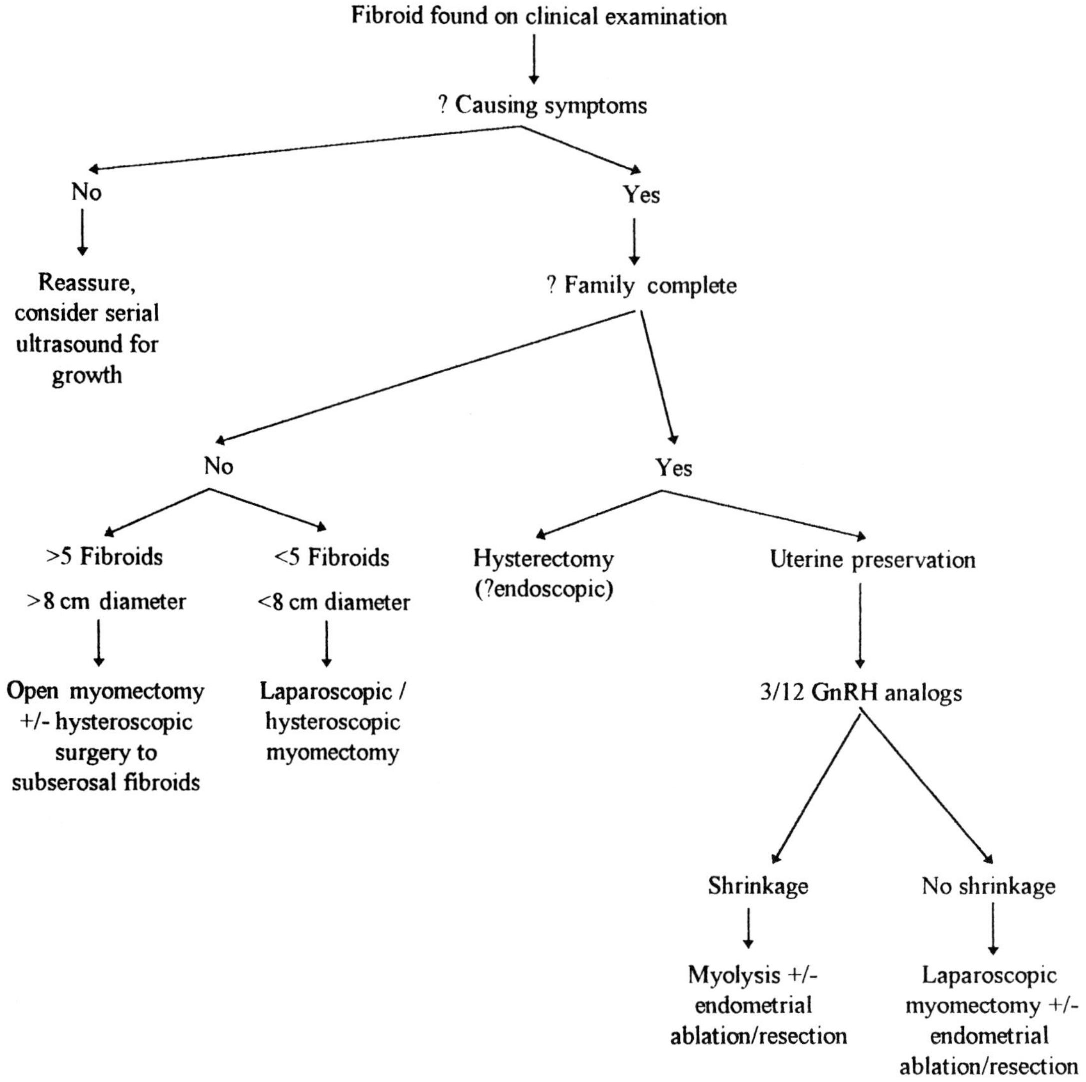

Figure flow chart:

Figure 5.3   An algorithm for management of uterine fibroids.

cern is the lack of tissue for histology although the risk of sarcomatous degeneration appears to be low at 0.04–0.29% of surgically removed fibroids (Montague *et al.*, 1965).

CONCLUSIONS

It is no longer necessary for women with symptomatic fibroids to have to undergo hysterectomy or open myomectomy in all cases. As with traditional surgery, the endoscopic treatment of fibroids will still depend on the number, site, size, growth rate of the fibroids and the symptoms caused and also the age, reproductive status and desires of the woman. Figure 5.3 shows an algorithm of suggested management for a woman found to have one or more fibroids on clinical examination. As for many other endoscopic procedures, long-term follow-up data on the treatment of fibroids will be needed if these techniques are to be accepted by the wider gynecological community.

REFERENCES

Baggish, M.S. and Daniell, J.F. (1989) Death caused by air embolism associated with nèodymium: yttrium-aluminium-garnet laser surgery and artificial sapphire tips. *Am J Obstet Gynecol*, **161**, 877–8.

Broadbent, J.A.M. and Magos, A.L. (1995) Menstrual blood loss after hysteroscopic myomectomy. *Gynaecol Endosc*, **4**, 41–4.

Brookes, P.G. (1996) Use of the vaporizing electrode during resectoscopic surgery. Paper presented at the *World Congress of Hysteroscopy*, Miami, 9–11 February.

Buttram, V.C. and Reiter, R.C. (1981) Uterine leiomyomata: aetiology, symptomatology and management. *Fertil Steril*, **36**, 433–45.

Candiani, G.B., Fedele, L., Parazzini, F. and Villa, L. (1991) Risk of recurrence after myomectomy. *Br J Obstet Gynaecol*, **98**, 385–9.

Daniell, J.F. and Gurley, L.D. (1991) Laparoscopic treatment of clinically significant symptomatic uterine fibroids. *J Gynaecol Surg*, **7**, 37–40.

Davids, A. (1952) Myomectomy: surgical technique and results in a series of 1150 cases. *Am J Obstet Gynecol*, **63**, 592–604.

Donnez, J. (1993) Nd:YAG laser hysteroscopic myomectomy, in *Endoscopic Surgery for Gynaecologists*, (eds. C.J.G. Sutton and M. Diamond), W.B. Saunders, London, pp. 327–30.

Donnez, J., Schrurs, B., Gillerot, S., Sandow, J. and Clercks, F. (1989) Treatment of uterine fibroids with implants of gonadotrophin-releasing hormone agonists: assessment by hysterography. *Fertil Steril*, **51**, 947.

Dubuisson, J.B. and Chapron, C. (1995) Laparoscopic myomectomy and myolysis, in *Baillières Clinical Obstetrics and Gynaecology. Advanced Laparoscopic Surgery*, (guest ed. C.J.G. Sutton), Baillière Tindall, London, pp. 717–28.

Dubuisson, J.B., Chavet, X., Chapron, C. and Morice, P. (1995) Uterine rupture during pregnancy after laparoscopic myomectomy. *Human Reprod*, **10**, 1475–7.

Filicori, M., Hall, D.A., Loughlin, J.S. *et al.* (1983) A conservative approach to the management of uterine leiomyomata: pituitary desensitization by a luteinizing hormone-releasing hormone analogue. *Am J Obstet Gynecol*, **147**, 726–7.

Gallinat, A. (1995) Myolysis. *Gynaecol Endosc*, **4**, 3–4.

Goldfarb, H.A. (1992) Nd:YAG laser laparoscopic coagulation of symptomatic myomas. *J Reprod Med*, **37**, 636–8.

Hamou, J. (1993) Electroresection of fibroids, in *Endoscopic Surgery for Gynaecologists*, (eds C.J.G. Sutton and M. Diamond), W.B. Saunders, London, pp. 327–30.

Harris, W.J. (1992) Uterine dehiscence following laparoscopic myomectomy. *Obstet Gynaecol*, **80**, 545–6.

Hasson, H.M., Rotman, C., Rana, N. *et al.* (1992) Laparoscopic myomectomy. *Obstet Gynaecol*, **80**, 884–8.

Manhes, H. and Lesec, G. (1988) Strategie combinee opposable aux leiomyomes ou myolyse. *Contraception, Fertilite, Sexualite*, **16**, 959–62.

Matta, W.H.M., Stabile, I., Shaw, R.S. and Campbell, S. (1988) Doppler assessment of uterine blood flow changes in patients with fibroids receiving the gonadotrophin-releasing hormone agonist buserelin. *Ferti Steril*, **49**, 1083–5.

McLucas, B. (1992) Diathermy polyp snare: a new modality for treatment of submucous myomata. *J Gynaecol Endosc*, **1**, 107–10.

Montague, A., Schwaetz, A. and Woodruff, J. (1965) Sarcoma arising in a leiomyoma of the uterus. *Am J Obstet Gynecol*, **92**, 421–7.

Myomectomy Adhesion Multicenter Study Group (1995) An expanded polytetrafluoroethylene barrier (Gore-Tex Surgical Membrane) reduces post-myomectomy adhesion formation. *Fertil Steril*, **63**, 491–3.

National Center for Health Statistics, Pokras, R. and Hufnagal, V.G. (1987) Hysterectomies in the United States, 1965–1984. *Vital and Health Statistics*. Series 13, No. 92. Government Printing Office, Washington DC.

Neuwirth, R.S. (1978) A new technique for and additional experience with hysteroscopic resection of submucous fibroids. *Am J Obstet Gynecol*, **131**, 91–4.

Neuwirth, R.S. and Amin, H.K. (1976) Excision of submucous fibroids with hysteroscopic control. *Am J Obstet Gynecol*, **126**, 95–9.

Nezhat, C., Nezhat, F., Silfen, S. *et al.* (1991) Laparoscopic myomectomy. *Int J Fertil*, **36**, 275–80.

Nezhat, C., Nezhat, F., Bess, O. *et al.* (1994) Laparoscopically assisted myomectomy: a report of a new technique in 57 cases. *Int J Fertil Menopausal Studies*, **39**, 39–44.

Nisolle, M., Smets, M., Malvaux, V. *et al.* (1993) Laparoscopic myolysis with the Nd:YAG laser. *J Gynaecol Surg*, **9**, 95–9.

Philips, D.R. (1995) Laparoscopic leiomyoma co-agulation (myolysis). *Gynaecol Endosc*, **4**, 5–12.

Semm, K. and Metler, L. (1980) Technical progress in pelvic surgery via operative laparoscopy. *Am J Obstet Gynecol*, **138**, 121.

Smith, C.J. (1952) Hysterectomy for benign pelvic conditions. *Am J Obstet Gynecol*, **64**, 1211–20.

Tulandi, T., Murray, C. and Guralnick, M. (1993) Adhesion formation and reproductive outcome after myomectomy and second-look laparoscopy. *Obstet Gynaecol*, **82**, 213–15.

Wamsteker, K. (1984) Hysteroscopy in the management of abnormal uterine bleeding in 199 patients, in *Hysteroscopy, Principles and Practice*, (eds A.M. Siegler and H.J. Lindemann), J.B. Lippincott, Philadelphia, pp. 128–31.

Wamsteker, K. (1993) Resection of intrauterine fibroids, in *Endometrial Ablation*, (eds B.V. Lewis and A.L. Magos), Churchill Livingstone, London, pp. 161–70.

LAPAROSCOPIC SURGERY FOR DYSMENORRHEA: UTERINE NERVE ABLATION AND PRESACRAL NEURECTOMY

E.D. Biggerstaff III and S.N. Foster

INTRODUCTION

Pelvic pain is one of the most common complaints addressed in gynecological practice. The etiology of pain may be simple and the location specific or the pain may be multifactorial in origin and diffuse in location. The pain may be affected by any number of physiological events including ovulation, menstruation, urination, digestion, defecation and coitus. It may be the patient's sole concern or there may be other considerations such as infertility. The severity and potential long-term sequelae of the pain must be considered when determining treatment alternatives. The scope of this discussion is not meant to address all aspects of pelvic pain, but a general discussion is necessary to assure appropriate selection of a therapeutic modality for a particular patient. A more detailed presentation on pelvic pain can be found in Bonica's (1990) text, *The Management of Pain*.

A number of conditions of either obstetric/gynecologic origin or non-obstetric/gynecologic origin can cause pain. These can include physiologic, traumatic, metabolic, infectious, neoplastic, non-neoplastic, and iatrogenic conditions. The actual insult that causes the transmission of impulses through the afferent (pain) neurons may be inflammatory, mechanical, ischemic or a combination of all three. Inflammation may result from an infectious process, chemical irritation or other sources such as endometriosis. Mechanical pain impulses arise when there is immobilization, obstruction, distention and/or contraction of a structure, viscus or organ. Finally, ischemia may play a part or be the sole agent in the production of pelvic pain.

The female pelvis is bounded by musculoskeletal structures and contains the pelvic viscera including the urinary bladder, the terminal portions of the ureters, a few loops of small intestine and frequently the appendix, the sigmoid colon and rectum, the uterus, fallopian tubes and ovaries along with their supporting ligaments and numerous blood vessels, lymph vessels and nodes and nerves. Any of these structures, individually or in combination with one another, can be the anatomic origin of pelvic pain. Additionally, pelvic pain may be totally or partially of psychosomatic etiology.

Pain may be located in the central pelvis, may be unilateral or bilateral or may arise from any combination of these sites. Midline pain usually arises from the uterus (including the cervix), uterosacral ligaments or the posterior cul-de-sac. Lateral pain arises more of-

Gynecological Endoscopic Surgery. Edited by C.J.G. Sutton. Published in 1997 by Chapman & Hall, London. ISBN 0 412 58040 3.

ten from the fallopian tubes, ovaries or lateral peritoneum (or other visceral structures noted above). Pain may radiate to the lower back, down one or both legs or to a combination of these locations.

To complete any discussion of pelvic pain, it is important to consider referred pain. It has been shown by McCoy and Bradford (1963) that afferent (pain) impulses arising from the viscera travel to the interneurons of the dorsal horn, which also receives impulses from the skin. This conversion of impulses from both cutaneous and visceral sources is most likely the mechanism of referred pain. Disease processes originating in the uterus, fallopian tubes or ovaries may result in perceived pain in any area of the anterior abdominal wall. Referred pain from the ovaries is also frequently perceived in the sacral area in the form of low back pain.

HISTORY

Physicians have used presacral neurectomy (PSN) to successfully treat women experiencing midline pelvic pain, intractable primary dysmenorrhea or dysmenorrhea secondary to endometriosis for almost 100 years (Fontaine and Herrmann, 1932; Davis, 1933; Cotte, 1937; Black, 1964). During the first 70 years of its use in treating women with midline pelvic pain and dysmenorrhea, the effectiveness of PSN was described in a series of case reports. Fontaine and Herrmann (1932) reported case histories of 22 women with functional dysmenorrhea and hypogastric plexalgia. All but two patients reported immediate relief from pain and 13 patients who were followed 'for a long period of time' after treatment with PSN reported no pain at follow-up. Counsellor and Craig (1934) reported the results of using PSN to treat 14 women with dysmenorrhea. Six women received only PSN and eight received treatment for pelvic lesions in addition to PSN. Twelve of the patients reported 100% relief and two reported 75% relief following the PSN. Cotte (1937) claimed that he had treated

almost 300 patients in 12 years with PSN and that only two had not experienced relief from pain following the procedure. Black (1964) summarized case reports from the literature (differentiating between treatment of primary and secondary dysmenorrhea) and calculated an 'overall success rate' of 79% for previously reported studies. He surveyed 800 physicians (472 responded) and 43 of his former patients who had been treated with PSN at least ten years prior to his study. The physician responses showed a 75% 'success rate' for patients' pain relief following treatment with PSN. Eighty percent of Dr Black's former patients were pain free ten or more years after treatment for primary or secondary dysmenorrhea with PSN. The literature and the patient survey reflected a slightly higher percentage of success for pain relief when treating primary dysmenorrhea, while the physicians' responses showed a small advantage when treating secondary dysmenorrhea or when the type of dysmenorrhea was not differentiated.

Doyle (1955) described a procedure for paracervical uterine denervation by transection of the cervical plexus. He emphasized the need to perform the transection 'as close to the uterus as possible' (p. 11), thus eliminating the need for an additional presacral neurectomy. He reported an 86% success rate for complete relief and a 95% success rate for complete or partial relief of pelvic pain in 73 patients followed from four months to four years postoperatively. Lichten and Bombard (1987) described a laparoscopic approach to Doyle's procedure. However, they reported that over 50% of the subjects treated with laparoscopic uterosacral nerve ablation (LUNA) in a double-blind study perceived the same or a greater level of pain 12 months postoperatively. Sutton (1992) reported an 84% success rate in pain relief two years postoperatively in 126 women with endometriosis or dysmenorrhea and suggested that advances in laparoscopic surgery may make Doyle's procedure more attractive to physicians treating patients for pelvic pain. Gürgan *et al.* (1992) used LUNA to treat 20 patients with primary dysmenorrhea. Fourteen of the women were seen for follow-up after one year. Eight of these subjects (57%) required medication for pain during menstrual periods and only five were free of significant pain (one additional patient was pregnant).

Introduction of the oral contraceptive pill (OCP) in the early 1960s had a major impact on the treatment of dysmenorrhea, as has the subsequent widespread use of prostaglandin synthetase inhibitors (PGSIs). Kistner (1979) introduced the concept of pseudo-pregnancy regimens using continuous combination OCPs when cyclic OCPs failed to relieve pain and dysmenorrhea due to endometriosis or at least presumably due to endometriosis. The symptoms frequently improve, but only transiently, especially when endometriosis is present. PGSIs, taken on a regular basis, especially prior to onset of symptoms, are effective for many women in relieving dysmenorrhea. Danazol was a mainstay in medical therapy of pain and dysmenorrhea associated with endometriosis (Greenblatt *et al.*, 1971), but Fedele *et al.* (1989) reported that over 90% of subjects treated with danazol experienced recurrence of endometriosis symptoms one year after stopping treatment. Gonadotropin-releasing hormone (GnRH) analogs were described as treatment by 'medical oophorectomy' for endometriosis by Meldrum and colleagues (1982), but Fedele and colleagues (1993) found a 42% recurrence rate of pain symptoms within one year of cessation of treatment of pelvic pain with buserelin acetate. The side effects of both groups of drugs are well known, as is the fact that the medications are expensive and require six months of therapy. Medical suppression will decrease the size of the lesions of endometriosis and diminish or eliminate pain, but the lesions remain and respond to cyclic hormonal stimulation when therapy is discontinued (Steingold *et al.*, 1987).

In recent years, the selection of PSN as an intervention for midline pain or dysmenorrhea usually followed unsuccessful treatment of the pain using oral contraceptives, nonsteroidal anti-inflammatory drugs (NSAIDs) and, in some cases, narcotics, as well as conservative surgical procedures such as laparoscopic resection of endometriosis and adhesions. Recent developments in laparoscopic surgery have enabled physicians to perform PSN laparoscopically, in conjunction with other conservative surgical procedures for the treatment of endometriosis or pelvic pain.

Perez (1990) reported the results of the first 25 cases that he treated with laparoscopic presacral neurectomy (LPSN). Using a ten-point pain scale, the patients rated the severity of their symptoms before and after undergoing LPSN. The patients reported a significant decrease in their pain symptoms postoperatively and they experienced no significant side effects following the procedure.

Nezhat and Nezhat (1992) performed a retrospective investigation of 52 patients from 1990–1992 who underwent LPSN for treatment of midline pain. They concurred with previous reports (Cotte, 1937; Doyle, 1955; Polan and DeCherney, 1980; Rock and Jones, 1983; Perez, 1990; Candiani *et al.*, 1992) that PSN significantly reduces midline pelvic pain and pain associated with intractable primary dysmenorrhea or secondary dysmenorrhea, but has little effect on adnexal pain. They recommended, as have others, that physicians carefully select patients for PSN or LPSN and that only those patients who have previously attempted medical therapy without relief of midline pain are candidates for the procedure (Fontaine and Herrmann, 1932; Counsellor and Craig, 1934; Black, 1964; Mahfoud and Hewitt, 1981; Fliegner and Umstad, 1991; Hill and Maher, 1991; Daniell *et al.*, 1993).

Perry and Perez (1993) continued implementation of the investigation previously undertaken by Perez (1990) and reported successful results in most of the 103 women treated with LPSN for midline suprapubic pelvic pain or dysmenorrhea. Eleven of the women treated with LPSN in this follow-up study had previously undergone laparoscopic uterosacral nerve ablation (LUNA) without relief of pelvic pain, but they all experienced alleviation of midline pain following the LPSN procedure. Perry and Perez reiterate the caution regarding careful patient selection and note, as have others (Davis, 1993; Cotte, 1937; Black, 1964; Beecham, 1978; Mahfoud and Hewitt, 1981; Fliegner and Umstad, 1991), that the most common reason for failure of LPSN to alleviate midline pelvic pain and dysmenorrhea is the incomplete resection of the presacral nerve.

More recently, Daniell *et al.* (1993) compared the results of laparoscopic presacral neurectomy using conventional retroperitoneal dissection techniques, lasers or sutures, with the results of laparoscopic presacral neurotomy using an argon beam coagulator (ABC) for tissue coagulation and separation. They found essentially no difference in the success rates (73% to 75%) between the two procedures. In addition, they reported the repair, by laparotomy, of an accidental laceration of the left common iliac vein, caused by the ABC beam. They, too, concluded that PSN should be attempted only after medical therapy and other conservative surgical intervention had failed and described PSN/LPSN as a last conservative intervention prior to using extirpative procedures for pain relief.

INDICATIONS FOR PRESACRAL NEURECTOMY

In recent years, medical therapy (especially with OCPs and PGSIs) has significantly reduced the need for surgical intervention when treating primary dysmenorrhea. Many cases of pelvic pain have specific etiologies amenable to medical therapy, such as infection or irritable bowel syndrome, and should be treated appropriately. LPSN is indicated for treatment of severe midline pelvic pain including dysmenorrhea which does not respond to medical or other appropriate therapy.

Dysmenorrhea is derived from Greek terms: *dys*, signifying painful or difficult; *men*, meaning smooth; and *rhein*, meaning to flow. Primary dysmenorrhea has no specific pathologic etiology but is felt to be associated with increased uterine muscular activity in response to increased prostaglandin production. Secondary dysmenorrhea, on the other hand, may have one of several origins: endometriosis, adenomyosis or the presence of an intrauterine device. Since the treatment of endometriosis is covered in great detail elsewhere in this book, no attempt will be made to duplicate this information but special mention should be made of adenomyosis.

Adenomyosis was first described by Cullen (1908) as a deep proliferation of normal endometrium. It is well known that adenomyosis may cause menorrhagia and dysmenorrhea or that it may be totally asymptomatic and that it is often found in association with uterine myomata as an incidental finding at pathological examination (Bird *et al.*, 1956; Bird and Molitor, 1971). Dysmenorrhea in association with the so-called 'boggy uterus' is often characteristic of adenomyosis with deep penetration of the uterus (Bird *et al.*, 1972). In a recent study, Nishida (1991) presented data suggesting that dysmenorrhea is directly related to the amount and size of the areas of adenomyosis in addition to the extent of the muscle invasion. He also noted a low incidence of dysmenorrhea in patients with adenomyotic lesions only on the serosal surface of the uterus when compared to those who had lesions extending from the endometrium.

Most authors concur that PSN significantly reduces midline pelvic pain and pain associated with intractable primary dysmenorrhea or secondary dysmenorrhea, but has little effect on lateral pain. In most cases there is general agreement that surgical intervention should be considered only after failure of medical therapy. One exception to this rule may be pain associated with infertility when known or suspected endometriosis is the culprit. In this case primary surgical intervention (not necessarily with PSN) is appropriate since medical suppression would simply delay the ability to conceive and not significantly improve the fecundity rate (Olive and Martin, 1987). In addition to unsuccessful medical therapy, many physicians reserve PSN for those patients who have also had failure of prior conservative surgical treatment including ablation of endometriosis and lysis of adhesions. In the authors' recent study of 28 patients (Biggerstaff and Foster, 1994), the potential benefits of using PSN as an initial surgical procedure to alleviate significant midline pain are presented. In combination with appropriate ablation of endometriosis and lysis of adhesions, primary PSN may prevent the need for additional surgical intervention for pain relief.

With the evolution of advanced endoscopic procedures including LPSN (Perez, 1990), the ability to treat a patient using minimally invasive surgical techniques has completely changed the implications of surgery when compared to traditional laparotomy and this change in implications for the patient may have a direct bearing on appropriate indications. If a procedure such as PSN requires laparotomy along with its accompanying recovery time and expense, all other avenues for therapy should be exhausted before proceeding. On the other hand, if PSN may be performed laparoscopically, why require the patient who has significant midline pain to come back for another procedure necessitating an additional anesthetic and expense when the procedure could be performed at the time of the initial ablation of the endometriosis?

Any discussion of indications for a particular procedure should also address the qualifications and skills of the surgeon planning to perform it. It is well recognized that the learning curve for laparoscopic procedures is longer than for the same procedures performed at laparotomy. A surgeon should demonstrate proficiency in performing a procedure at laparotomy prior to performing it laparoscopically and must be able to manage any associated complications should they arise. Because of the anatomical area in which PSN is performed, there may be a greater likelihood of significant complication in PSN than with most gynecological procedures unless meticulous dissection technique is maintained. Without appropriate training and/or skills, it is best that a surgeon either refer a patient to a surgeon with this ability to safely perform the procedure or consider another appropriate treatment, if that alternative exists.

ANATOMY

A thorough understanding of the relevant anatomy is vital to performing a procedure which is both safe and complete. It is also important to realize that the relative location of several structures including the sigmoid colon, certain vessels, the ureters and nerve plexus itself may vary considerably.

The so-called 'presacral nerve' (Figure 6.1) is found in a triangular area known as the interiliac trigone (Elaut, 1933). The lower limit of the trigone is the sacral promontory and the lateral boundaries are formed by the common iliac arteries meeting at the bifurcation of the aorta above. The right ureter is usually seen at the lateral limit of the dissection as it crosses the common iliac artery, just prior to or at its bifurcation into the external iliac and hypogastric vessels. The corresponding veins course under the arteries. On the left side there is most often a similar positional relationship between the ureter and the common iliac artery on that side.

The dissection on the left side is not commonly carried far enough laterally to visualize the ureter. Since the ureter on the left side may occasionally be seen more medially than described, care must be taken during dissection to avoid damaging this structure. The usual limits of dissection on the left side are the infe-

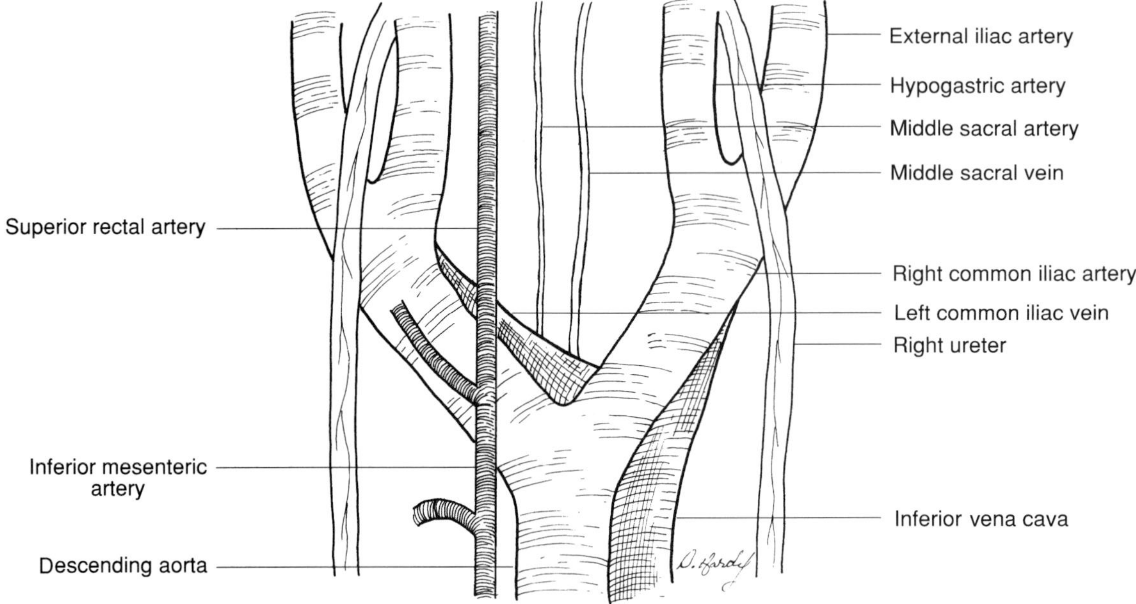

Figure 6.1   Anatomy in the area of the interiliac trigone (actual view as obtained on laparoscopy).

rior mesenteric artery and the base of the sigmoid mesocolon. The inferior mesenteric artery arises approximately 4 cm above the bifurcation, then descends in front of and finally alongside the left side of the aorta. At the level of the left common iliac artery, the inferior mesenteric artery splits into several branches. It continues into the pelvis as the superior rectal (hemorrhoidal) artery and branches laterally into the left colic and 2–4 sigmoid arteries. During presacral neurectomy, caution must be exercised to avoid damage to the left common iliac vein since it runs much more medially than the artery and actually forms a portion of the trigone floor on this side.

Embryologically the middle sacral artery is a continuation of the aorta. The middle sacral artery is a very thin vessel that arises from the posterior aspect of the aorta (before it bifurcates) and continues over the fourth and fifth lumbar vertebrae, the sacrum and the coccyx. The middle sacral vein, which can be a significant source of blood loss if damaged, arises

from the left common iliac vein and parallels the path of the middle sacral artery.

The lower colon, bladder and pelvic organs have an abundant nerve supply arising from the thoracic, lumbar and sacral levels of the spinal cord. There are both afferent (or sensory) and efferent (or sympathetic and parasympathetic) components. Sensory innervation of the lower uterine segment and cervix was previously thought to be supplied by sacral segments (Head, 1893; Cleland, 1933). Most modern obstetric and anatomy textbooks still report this innervation path (Greenhill, 1965; Williams and Warwick, 1980; Clemente, 1985; Pritchard *et al.*, 1985). However, recent data form Bonica (1990) contradicts this assumption. Bonica's work demonstrates that the afferent supply of the entire uterus and proximal fallopian tubes accompanies other sympathetic nerves as follows (Figure 6.2). The uterine and cervical plexuses combine to form the pelvic plexus (ganglion of Frankenhauser) and on each side course posteriorly over the lateral surface of the

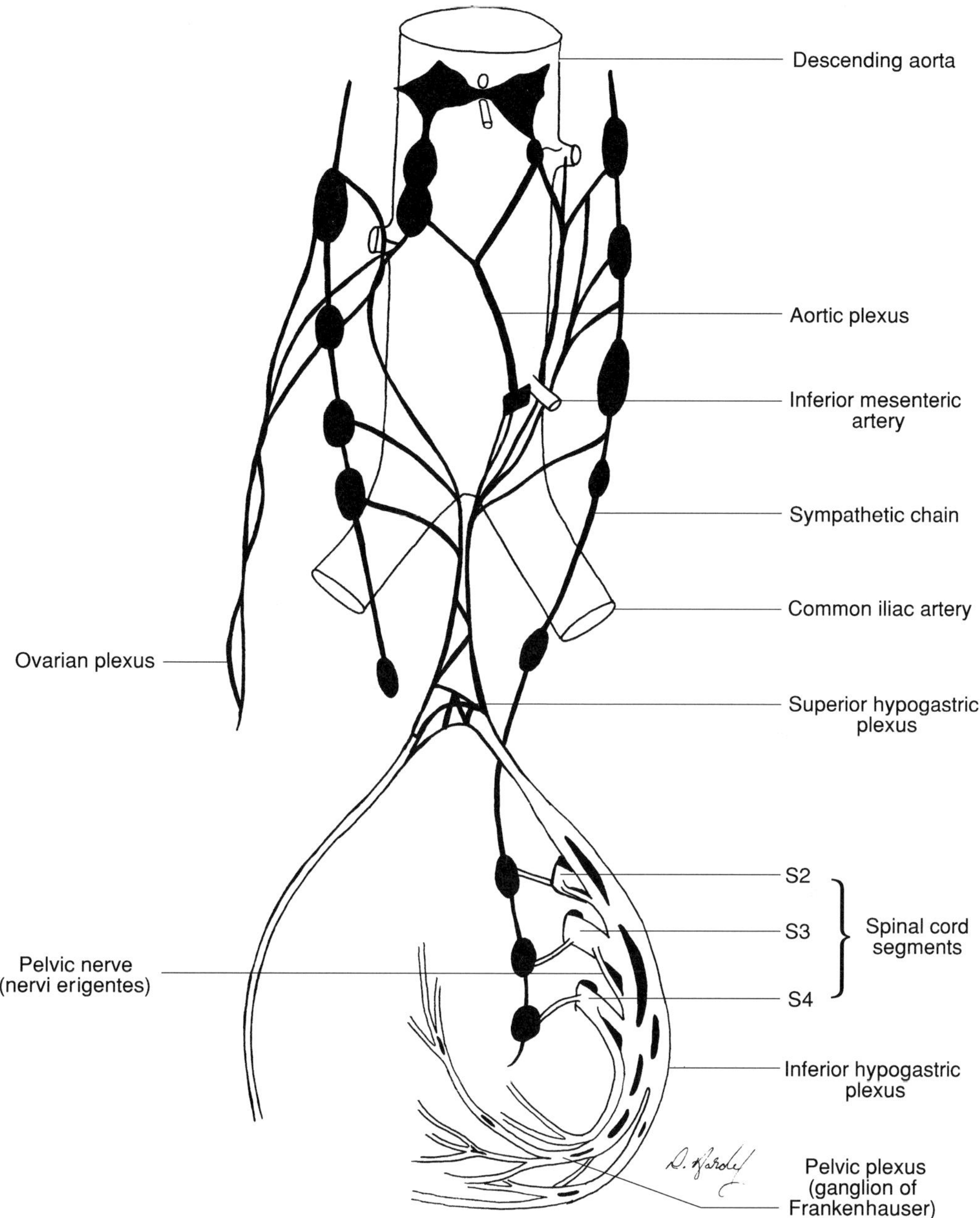

Figure 6.2   Nerve supply to the pelvis.

rectal ampulla. They then join the inferior hypogastric nerve plexuses near the sacral end of the uterosacral ligaments. Traveling cephalad, these plexuses form the middle hypogastric plexus, or hypogastric nerve, on either side just below the level of the sacral promontory.

The hypogastric nerve may be a single nerve

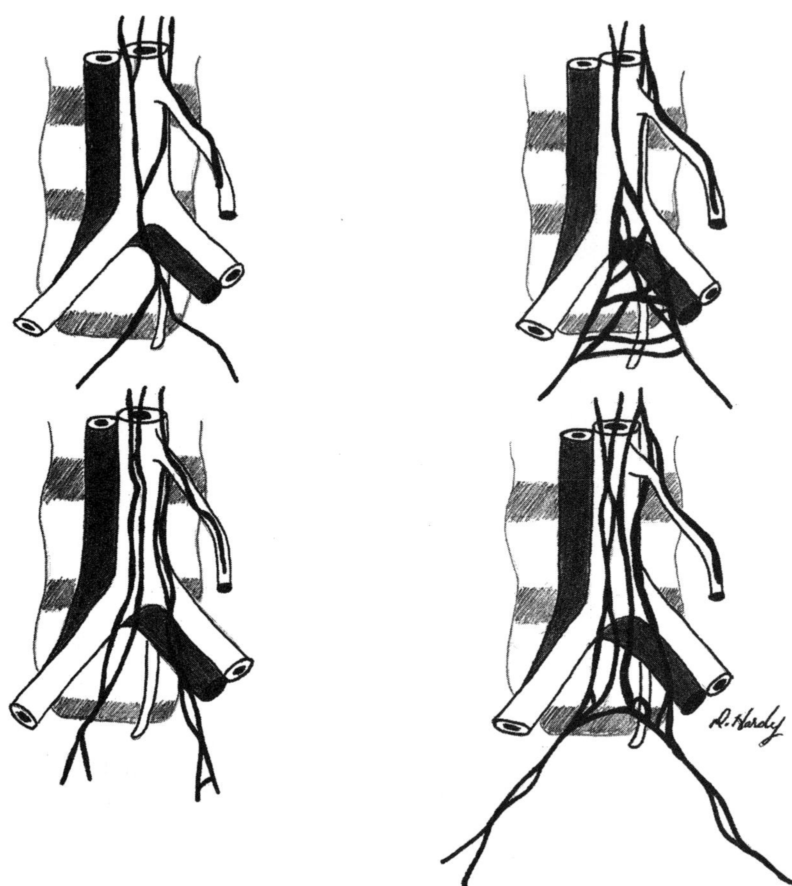

Figure 6.3   Different configurations of the superior hypogastric plexus.

or several fibers connected by anastomosing elements. This plexus becomes the superior hypogastric plexus or so-called 'presacral nerve'. A network of veins lies under the middle hypogastric plexus which can cause troublesome bleeding should they be damaged during surgery. The superior hypogastric plexus is in loose areolar tissue, overlying the sacral promontory and middle sacral vessels and under the peritoneum. The breadth of the plexus may vary considerably, as can the degree of condensation of fibers. Also, the plexus can be in multiple layers. In 20–25% of cases, a single nerve is found (Wharton, 1977). More often there are 2–4 incompletely fused nerve trunks in a broad, flat plexus (Figure 6.3). The plexus tends to be off center, more frequently

to the left. The superior hypogastric plexus leads to the aortic plexus. The afferent fibers course through the lumbar sympathetic chain and cephalad through the lower thoracic sympathetic chain. The fibers leave the chain via the rami communicantes of the T10, T11, T12 and L1 spinal nerves and go through the posterior roots to synapse with interneurons in the dorsal horn.

When considering treatment of pelvic pain, it is also important to recognize that the sensory nerve supply of the ovaries, distal fallopian tubes and posterior broad ligaments is separate from that of the uterus (Figure 6.2). The nerve fibers from these structures follow the same course as the ovarian vessels and terminate in the ovarian plexus on each side.

The ovarian plexuses arise from the aortic and renal plexus. The close proximity of the nerves and vascular supply prevents ovarian denervation from being a practical procedure.

Understanding the innervation of the remaining pelvic viscera (Figure 6.2) is important when considering interruption of nerves for treatment of pelvic pain and when considering other possible effects of this nerve interruption (Bonica, 1975; Renaer and Guzinski, 1978). The sympathetic nerve supply for the lower colon and rectum, in addition to the majority of that for the bladder, is derived from the sacral splanchnic nerves which in turn arise from the sacral portion of the sympathetic chain. A portion of the sympathetic nerve supply of the bladder also travels through the inferior, middle and superior hypogastric plexus. The parasympathetic supply for the lower colon, rectum and bladder comes mainly from direct branches of the pelvic splanchnic nerves originating in spinal cord segments S2, S3 and S4. Afferent fibers from the lower colon accompany the parasympathetic nerves and enter the spinal cord in the same segments. The sensory supply to the rectum is through the pudendal nerve, as is that to the external and internal vesicle sphincters and adjacent parts of the bladder. The peritoneum of the dome of the bladder is supplied by afferent fibers of the T11 to L1 spinal nerves.

ALTERNATIVE THERAPIES AND CONSIDERATIONS

Medical therapy for pelvic pain and dysmenorrhea has been presented briefly in prior sections and should be considered in most cases before proceeding with surgical intervention. Again, a notable exception to this is the patient who has unsuccessfully attempted conception and who has concomitant pain.

Paracervical uterine denervation as described by Doyle (1955), along with the LUNA procedure, have been promoted by many as an effective treatment for midline pelvic pain and dysmenorrhea. As noted previously, the long-term pain relief with these procedures is less than optimal. The authors agree with Malinak (1980), who states that the only indication for resection (or ablation) of the proximal uterosacral ligament is when pathology such as endometriosis or a myoma is present in this site.

Other pain-controlling techniques include injections of certain agents for nerve blockage or destruction, dilation and curettage, hymenotomy and various neurosurgical procedures. Different anesthetic agents or alcohol injected into Frankenhauser's plexus or other areas of afferent nerve supply from the pelvis have been used to try to alleviate pain (Evans, 1971). These injections are blind procedures which have unpredictable results and should not be used in the management of pelvic pain. More recently, computed tomography-guided neurolysis of the presacral and precoccygeal sympathetic trunk has been used on a limited basis to treat pelvic pain caused by tumor infiltration (mostly colorectal and gynecological carcinomas) of the pelvis (Seibel and Gronemeyer, 1990). Since the total number of patients on which this procedure has been performed is limited, this technique should be considered experimental at this time.

Any obstruction to the efflux of menstrual discharge may worsen or cause dysmenorrhea. The totally intact hymen and associated hematocolpometra is an unusual cause of cyclic midline pain, but one that lends itself to easy surgical correction in most cases. Dilation and curettage is rarely indicated as a therapeutic tool for dysmenorrhea, but dilation of a significantly stenotic cervix may improve or eliminate dysmenorrhea. Depending on the cause of the stenosis, the patient must be advised that the dilation may be only temporary and that the pain may return with recurrence of the stenosis. Hysteroscopy should be performed at the time of cervical dilation to look for evidence of adenomyosis. The diagnosis of adenomyosis is not an easy one to make at hysteroscopy and requires a careful scanning of the endometrial surface. If the lesions extend from the surface of the endometrium, one can visualize the ostia of the diverticula as dark depressions that vary in size. The openings may be obscured by the endometrium or may be seen just under the surface of the endometrium when they lie not too far from it (Barbot, 1989). Laparoscopy to ablate endometriosis, if present, along with presacral neurectomy, should be considered at the same time as cervical dilation for severe cervical stenosis, especially when adenomyosis is known or suspected. Several neurosurgical procedures including cordotomy, rhizotomy and myelotomy are used to treat severe pain associated with pelvic neoplasm but are not appropriate for the treatment of non-neoplastic pain.

'Definitive' surgical treatment for midline pelvic pain and dysmenorrhea traditionally has required hysterectomy, with or without the removal of the fallopian tubes and ovaries. Certain cases may lend themselves to a vaginal approach, including removal of the adnexa if desired. The authors recommend that this approach not be taken when the indication (or one of the indications) is significant pelvic pain because endometriosis may be left *in situ* and be a persistent source of pain. Of even greater potential consequence, endometriosis may be left and buried in the cuff at closure, making subsequent removal of the endometriosis more difficult. For these reasons, laparoscopically assisted vaginal hysterectomy is preferred over the vaginal approach to increase the likelihood of complete ablation of endometriosis if present.

The other question regarding definitive surgery is whether or not the ovaries should be removed at the time of hysterectomy. In a recent study, Namnoum and colleagues (1993) presented data suggesting that ovarian conservation at the time of hysterectomy increases the risk of persistence of symptoms when the surgery is performed to treat pain secondary to endometriosis. In a series of 147 women, 117 had all ovarian tissue removed while 30 had some preservation of ovarian tissue at the time of hysterectomy. Of those patients with no ovarian conservation, 7% had recurrent symptoms and 1.7% required reoperation for persistent symptomatology. With conservation of some ovarian function, 63% had recurrent symptoms and 30% required reoperation. In addition to recurrent pain, other factors such as the risk of developing ovarian cancer, other pelvic pathology (such as adhesions) and the psychological impact of oophorectomy must be considered and discussed with the patient. If the ovaries are not removed and there is subsequent need for oophorectomy, current technique will usually allow laparoscopic removal as an outpatient rather than requiring laparotomy, unless malignancy is present.

PREOPERATIVE EVALUATION AND THERAPY

The first step to successful outcome of any surgical procedure is thorough preoperative evaluation and preparation of the patient. A *current* medical history and physical examination are of the utmost importance. A number of factors must be taken into consideration before proceeding with surgical intervention. The patient's age, health status, weight and fertility desires all have a major bearing on whether a definitive procedure is appropriate (such as a hysterectomy with removal of fallopian tubes and ovaries) or whether a more conservative approach is desirable. Another consideration is the psychological/cultural impact of total pelvic clean-out. Even though fertility may not be desired by the patient, conservation of menstrual and endogenous hormonal function until the time of natural menopause is very important to many women and should be addressed during preoperative counseling. A complete history should also include questions regarding the possibility of childhood physical and sexual abuse, which have been shown to have a direct correlation with pelvic pain in women during adulthood (Walker *et al.*, 1988). The etiology of pelvic pain, in addition to other medical problems such as irritable bowel syndrome, may be an inability to tolerate 'normal' physical symptoms as a result of the childhood trauma. It has been shown that patients may experience anxiety and hyperarousal with respect to body sensation along with acute and chronic depression after sexual assault (Courtois, 1988; Herman, 1992). In this situation the origin of the patient's pain is physical, but the reaction and interpretation are psychological. Appropriate preoperative evaluation should rule out non-gynecologic causes of pain, assess the status of the pelvis prior to surgery and may include intravenous pyelography, barium enema, enhanced computed tomography, magnetic resonance imaging, etc.

Assessment should include a current dietary history in addition to a listing of both prescription and over-the-counter medications. The patient should not be on a weight reduction diet within two weeks of planned surgery due to possible coagulation problems and delayed healing. Also any medication containing aspirin or aspirin-like compounds should be avoided to reduce the likelihood of excessive bleeding.

Informed consent is a preoperative requirement in most areas throughout the United States. It has evolved as a formal tool to insure that the patient fully understands all aspects of the proposed surgery and to document this understanding in writing. The details of informed consent vary from state to state, but generally include the following:

- patient's name and date (generally must be dated within 30 days of the date of surgery);
- the diagnosis requiring the procedure;
- a request by the patient that the designated surgeon perform the specified procedure;
- a detailed description of the procedure;
- possible complications of the procedure;
- an assessment of the likelihood of success of the procedure;
- possible alternatives to the proposed procedure including both surgical and non-surgical alternatives;

- various disclaimers including the fact that 'no guarantees or assurances have been made to the patient';
- a signature block that acknowledges understanding and agreement to the contents of the consent form.

Preoperative therapy should include bowel preparation unless it is known from recent surgical evaluation that there is no bowel involvement with endometriosis or adhesions. Preoperative bowel preparation is becoming almost standard with all gynecological surgery, whether it is done at laparotomy or laparoscopy, since it seems to reduce the incidence of postoperative ileus and provides a margin of safety should the bowel be accidentally or intentionally entered. One regimen for bowel preparation includes two days of clear liquids until midnight before surgery, then nothing by mouth until surgery. Additionally, one gallon of Go-lytely™ (Lyne Laboratories) is consumed between 2 p.m. and 6 p.m. the day prior to surgery. The Go-lytely™ tastes like a salty soda water and is difficult for many patients to tolerate without significant emesis. Thorough explanation of the rationale for the bowel prep, along with the liberal use of mouthwash while drinking Go-lytely™ and placing the reconstituted solution in the refrigerator 24 hours ahead to allow it to become ice cold will frequently make oral consumption more tolerable. Finally, cefonicid sodium (Monocid, SK&F) 1 gram IV is given one hour prior to surgery to complete bowel preparation.

If the primary or assisting surgeons do not have the training or skills required to perform interoperative cystoscopy and gastrointestinal endoscopy, arrangements should be made preoperatively for these services to be available should they be required during any advanced laparoscopic procedure. When localization of the ureter is made difficult by adhesions, inflammatory reaction and endometriosis (Sackier, 1993) the illuminated 6 Fr ureteric probe (Karl Storz Endoscopy,

America) can be especially helpful. Gastrointestinal endoscopy can be utilized when there is a question regarding whether or not the mucosa of the bowel is intact.

PROCEDURE

Laparoscopic presacral neurectomy is performed under general anesthesia. The patient is placed in the low lithotomy position so that a uterine manipulator can be used to facilitate adequate endoscopic examination of the pelvis and assist in appropriate treatment of pelvic pathology when present. A four-puncture technique is preferred: an umbilical incision is made through which to insert a 10 mm operating laparoscope and three incisions made just below the pubic hair line for sleeves accommodating 5 mm instruments. A video camera with adequate resolution and color separation is attached to the laparoscope. An alternative to using an operating laparoscope is to use a purely diagnostic one. The diagnostic laparoscope has the obvious advantage of better illumination, whereas the laparoscope with an operating channel may be preferred if the carbon dioxide laser is chosen, along with other instruments, without needing an additional port for the laser or these instruments.

The first case in the authors' series of patients treated with laparoscopic presacral neurectomy was completed with the laparoscope inserted through a suprapubic midline incision looking cephalad (Biggerstaff and Foster, 1994). There was found to be no particular advantage to this approach and all cases since this initial one have been performed with the laparoscope inserted through an umbilical incision. For the lower incisions, one is made in the midline and the other two just lateral to the rectus muscles, taking care to avoid both the superficial and deep vessels of the abdominal wall. If monopolar electrocautery is to be used, conductive metal sleeves should be utilized through all incisions to minimize the chance of accidental injury to vital adjacent structures. The conductive

sleeves allow dispersion of electrical current throughout the entire abdominal wall and reduce the likelihood that an electrical arc will burn bowel or other adjacent structures. In order to further reduce the likelihood of electrical injury, in addition to lowering the cost of the procedure, non-disposable or reusable instruments are employed whenever possible. Also, it has been demonstrated that the insulation on many disposable instruments is inadequate in thickness to protect against electrical injury.

The laparoscopic presacral neurectomy is initiated after any other procedures necessary to treat pelvic disease are completed. The goal of surgical therapy for pelvic pain should be complete removal of all typical and atypical endometriosis and adhesions (Martin *et al.*, 1989) in addition to other procedures deemed appropriate, such as presacral neurectomy.

Various instruments can be used for the peritoneal incision and subsequent dissection, including the carbon dioxide (CO_2) laser, argon laser, potassium titanyl phosphate (KTP) laser, sapphire-tipped neodymium:yttrium aluminum garnet (Nd-YAG) laser, the argon beam coagulator, the harmonic scalpel, various mono- and bipolar electrical instruments and scissors. The surgeon should choose the instruments that he is most skilled with and be aware of the effects, potential dangers and limitations of each. Additionally, hemaclips and sutures are now used laparoscopically and may be appropriate when performing presacral neurectomy. Due to the vascularity of the area in addition to personal preference, the authors most commonly employ scissors with and without cutting current, in addition to bipolar cautery to control larger vessels. Blunt dissection may be carried out with various forceps, irrigation aspirators and scissors.

A transverse incision is made in the peritoneum overlying the sacral promontory, extending from the ureter on the right side to the inferior mesenteric and superior hemorrhoidal arteries and sigmoid colon on the left

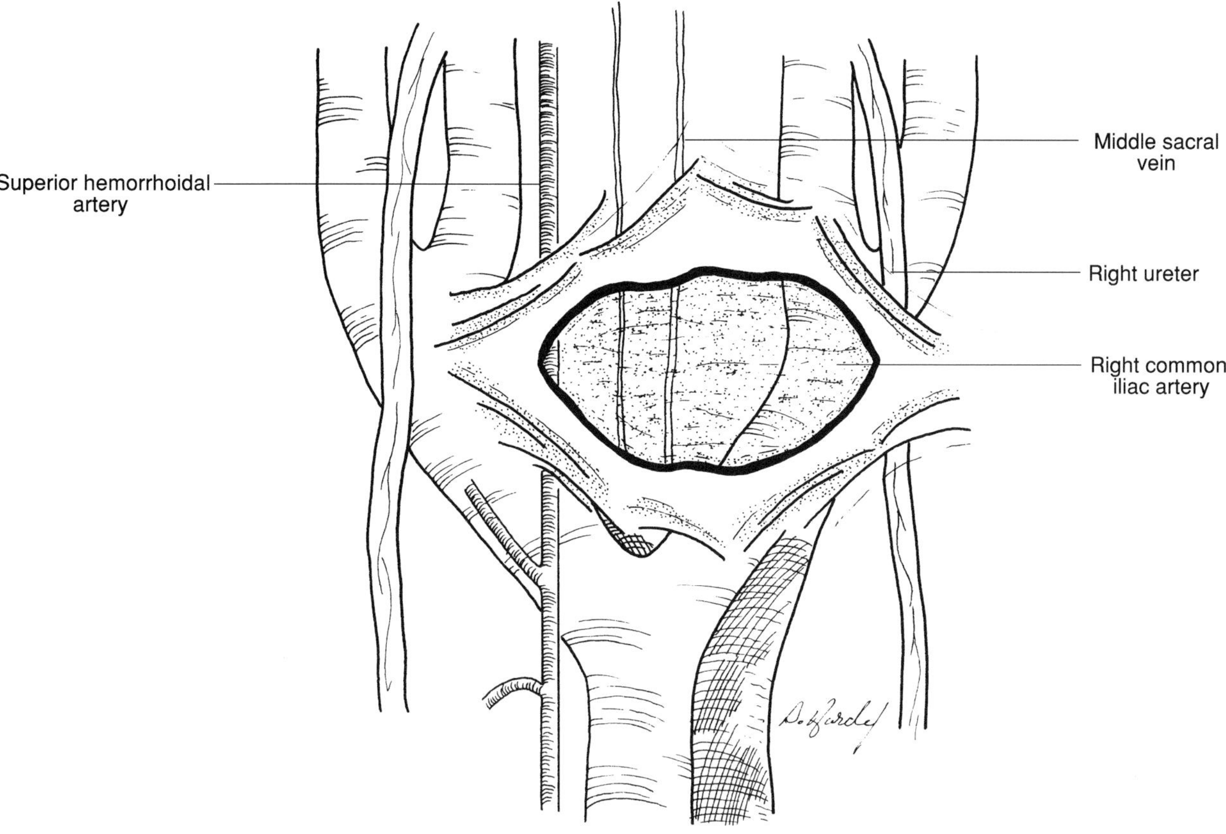

Figure 6.4 Transverse incision in peritoneum overlying sacral promontory (actual view as obtained on laparoscopy).

side (Figure 6.4). The landmarks on the right side are usually easily identifiable through the peritoneum, but not so on the left side. The inferior mesenteric and superior hemorrhoidal arteries are found in fatty connective tissue and may be difficult to locate. Additionally, care must be taken to avoid damage to the sigmoid colon itself. In a series of 28 cases (Biggerstaff and Foster, 1994), the left ureter was found within the limits of dissection only once; caution is necessary to avoid possible injury to this structure. The sigmoid colon must be retracted to a left lateral position to obtain adequate exposure for the presacral neurectomy. This is most easily accomplished with an atraumatic grasping forceps introduced through the left suprapubic sleeve which simultaneously elevates the left end of the incision and retracts the sigmoid colon.

When the limits of the dissection are difficult to identify (always on the left side), a 'T' incision should be used, beginning at the middle of the transverse incision in the peritoneum and carrying the incision cephalad to the bifurcation of the descending aorta and inferior vena cava (Figure 6.5). There is no advantage to exposing the operative field below the prominence of the sacrum since dissection in this area will very likely result in venous bleeding that is difficult to control. The dissection is usually begun on the right side and carried to the left. Connective and fatty tissue which contains the nerve plexus is dissected both sharply and bluntly and isolated in small

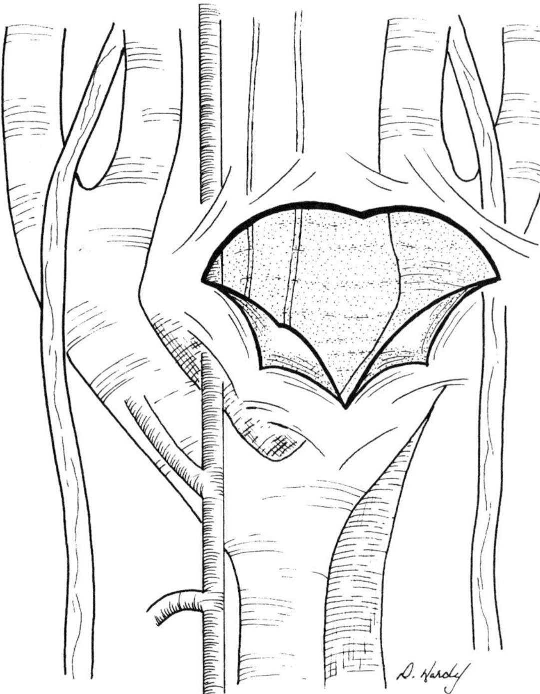

Figure 6.5 Transverse incision converted to 'T' incision (actual view as obtained on laparoscopy).

longitudinal bunches, cauterized in two places 1–2 cm apart, removed and sent to pathology to confirm removal of nerve elements (Figure 6.6). When the dissection is complete, the sacral promontory has the appearance of a 'baby's bottom', with the intact middle sacral vein running down the middle (Figure 6.7). Most gynecological surgeons leave the peritoneum open, realizing spontaneous reperitonealization will occur in a short period of time. If closure is desired, it can be accomplished either with staples or sutures.

Unless there are other reasons for overnight hospitalization, most patients may be discharged home when they are voiding and ambulatory after laparoscopic presacral neurectomy. Oral pain medication and an antiemetic are prescribed and the patient is seen within one week from surgery. Most patients are able to return to all but the most strenuous activities within a week and may resume sexual activity within several weeks.

COMPLICATIONS

Potential complications of LPSN include those which are common to all laparoscopic procedures and those which are unique to LPSN. This section will give a brief overview of those common to all laparoscopies and provide more detail regarding complications seen more often with presacral neurectomy. Although unusual, complications may be related to general anesthesia itself and may be accentuated by certain factors unique to laparoscopy. These factors are decreased diaphragmatic excursion secondary to pneumoperitoneum and steep Trendelenburg position; hypercarbia and possibly mild acidosis and arrhythmias associated with carbon dioxide use and decreased ventilatory capacity; and the possibility of decreased cardiac output due to intra-abdominal CO_2 pressure causing decreased venous return, especially in the older patient. Careful continuous monitoring of the patient's status by anesthesia personnel should avert most problems, but a slight change in the patient's position or decrease in intra-abdominal pressure may be required to maintain normal parameters.

More commonly, complications occur as a direct result of laparoscopy or as a result of procedures performed at the time of laparoscopy. Laceration of a viscus or blood vessel may occur at initial entry with the Veress needle, as can erroneous placement of the carbon dioxide gas. Especially with longer cases, subcutaneous emphysema may occur without erroneous placement when the gas leaks through the peritoneum around the various sleeves. A marked swelling of the mons pubis can result, but is rarely of any long-term consequence. Subcutaneous emphysema which has traveled cephalad has twice caused an unusual but inconsequential complication in the authors' experience, that of bleeding

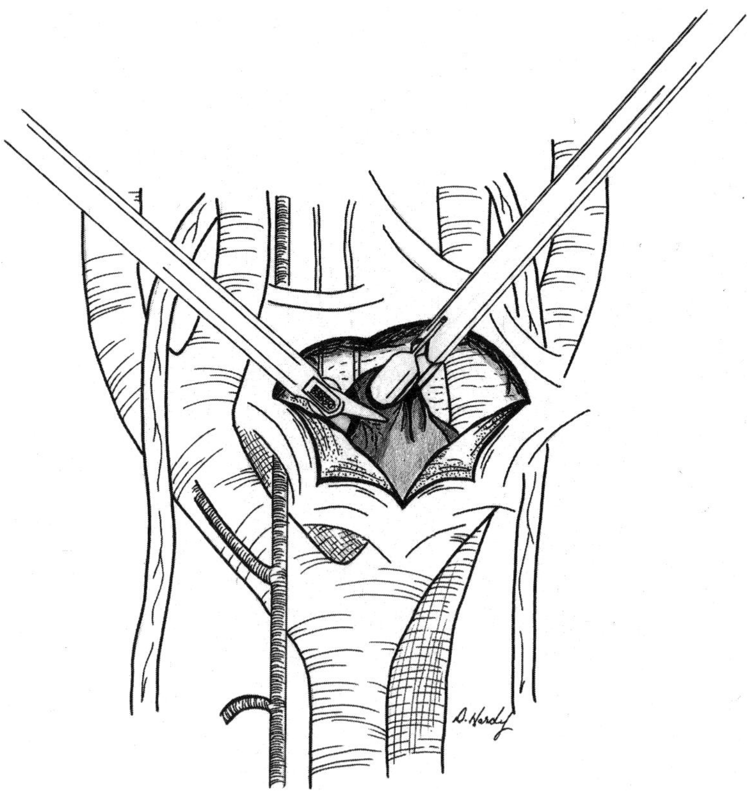

Figure 6.6 Removal of tissue over sacral promontory (actual view as obtained on laparoscopy).

from the ear noted at termination of the surgical case. Immediate examination by an otolaryngologist in both instances revealed small blebs of subcutaneous gas in the auditory canal with a site of bleeding easily controlled by packing and with no ill effect to the patient. Careful examination did demonstrate previously undetected subcutaneous emphysema.

Introduction of the laparoscopic sleeve and trocar as well as those for ancillary ports can also result in damage to internal organs or structures. Once the laparoscopic sleeve is in place, the structures under the insertion point should be carefully examined for any sign of damage. Pointing the laparoscope directly towards the patient's back will also help the surgeon identify laceration of a significant vessel within the umbilicus if one sees blood dripping on the omentum and bowel below. The Hassan cannula should be used with direct visualization of the initial entry whenever it is suspected that bowel or omentum may be adhered to the anterior abdominal wall. In spite of careful entry technique, inadvertent entry into the bowel may occasionally occur and can usually be repaired either while the bowel is still attached to the anterior wall or with laparoscopic suturing.

Injury may occur with any energy modality or instrument used at laparoscopy. The American Association of Gynecologic Laparoscopists conducted a survey (Peterson *et al.*, 1990) showing a serious complication rate of 1.54% in 36 928 procedures performed by 880 respondents. The most frequent complications were persistent elevated human chorionic gonadotropin titer after treatment of ectopic

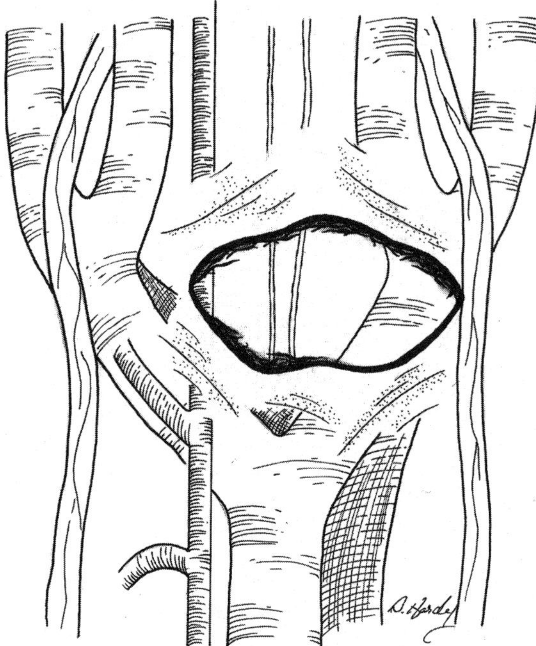

Figure 6.7 Appearance after completion of presacral neurectomy – note intact presacral vessels (actual view as obtained on laparoscopy).

pregnancy, hospital readmission and unintended laparotomy to treat bowel injury, urinary tract injury or hemorrhage.

Most serious long-term consequences are a result of a failure to identify and repair damage to a structure at the time of initial laparoscopy. If there is uncertainty regarding potential damage, liberal use of adjunctive endoscopy such as colonoscopy or cystoscopy with ureteral stents can help confirm or deny these suspicions.

Complications specific to LPSN are related to possible effects of cutting the 'presacral nerve' or superior hypogastric plexus and to the anatomical site where the procedure is performed. Meticulous dissection technique, along with knowledge of the relative anatomy and its possible variances, will help avoid most complications, including injury to the bowel, vessels and ureters. Along with dissection technique, the surgeon must have full knowledge of the limitations and potential hazards of the energy modalities being used.

The most significant intraoperative complication reported is hemorrhage, usually from the middle sacral vein or its branches, or from a larger vessel, most often the left common iliac vein. Interruption of the middle sacral vein or its companion artery can cause significant blood loss. Careful dissection can usually avoid damage to these relatively small vessels which can often be visualized through the peritoneum before the initial incision is made. If occlusion of either of these vessels is necessary, it can usually be accomplished with bipolar cautery or with a laparoscopically placed suture. An appropriate suture would be a 3-0 braided polyglycolic acid or silk suture on a small, curved, taper needle transfixed to the periostium. Placing the suture through the periostium decreases the likelihood of tearing the vessel and its branches which will result in further bleeding. Pastner and Orr (1990) reported the use of stainless steel thumbtacks to control intractable venous hemorrhage at the time of conventional PSN. Several small branches of the presacral venous plexus were lacerated and could not be controlled with bovie cautery, suture ligation, packing with bone wax or attempted collusion with hemaclips. LPSN offers the distinct advantage over conventional PSN of close visual proximity with magnification, which should decrease the chance of accidental laceration of these vessels. If the dissection is either begun or carried just below the sacral promontory, bleeding from the venous plexus in this location is significantly increased.

The left common iliac vein is the large vessel most often reported to be damaged at LPSN. The vessel frequently runs more medially than anticipated and actually forms a lateral portion of the floor of the interiliac trigone. If there is uncertainty regarding the location of this vessel or of any structure, the initial transverse incision in the peritoneum overlying the sacral promontory should be converted to a 'T' incision as previously described (Figure 6.5).

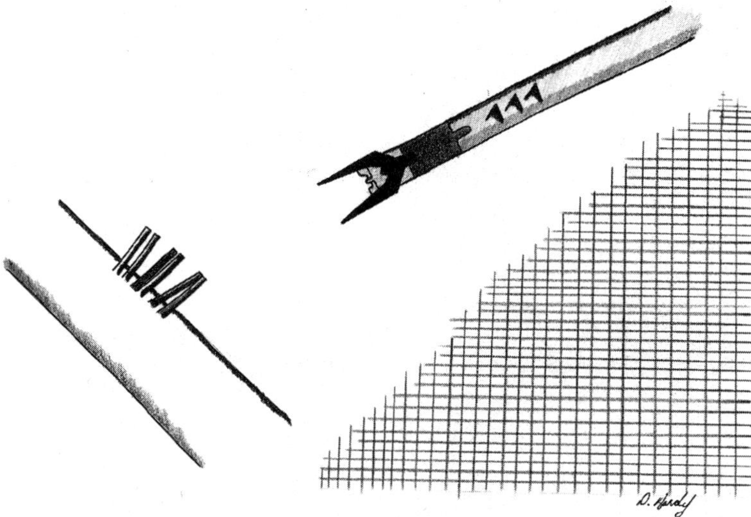

Figure 6.8 Repair of large vessel laceration with hemaclips.

Laceration of the left common iliac vein has required laparotomy for repair, usually with significant blood loss requiring blood transfusion. The authors recently reported (Biggerstaff and Foster, 1994) laparoscopic repair of this vessel using a series of hemaclips. During dissection on the left side of the interiliac trigone, an area of tissue, when lifted, was noted to have a slight bluish tinge. This appearance is not unusual when cutting through connective tissue. Rather than continuing with the dissection, conversion to a 'T' incision would have enabled accurate identification of the structure. A 1 cm incision was made with scissors and venous blood immediately obscured the operative field. In order to repair the vessel, it was quickly grasped where the laceration occurred with a smooth forceps and gently lifted to stop the bleeding. Adequate exposure and a dry field are mandatory for successful laparoscopic repair in this situation. Additional instrument ports may be necessary, as will a 10 mm suction instrument. Once the bleeding was temporarily stopped, the laparotomy set was opened, type and crossmatch of blood was begun and consultation with a vascular surgeon took place. A row of parallel hemaclips (Figure 6.8) was used to close the laceration with the method agreed upon with the consulting vascular surgeon. An alternative method for closure is the use of precise intracorporeal suturing and knot-tying techniques, performed in a manner similar to that at laparotomy.

The closure with hemaclips described above caused a compromise of less than a quarter of the diameter of the vessel and the resultant blood loss was less than 50 cc. If it is possible to immediately grasp and occlude the vessel, the patient will be likely to lose less blood than if one proceeds to immediate laparotomy. If the bleeding cannot be controlled laparoscopically, laparotomy should be performed without hesitation. The temptation to grasp a large vessel with a bipolar cautery instrument and apply electrical current should always be avoided. This will inevitably result in a larger hole in the vessel than the initial one. Prevention of accidental laceration of vessels at laparoscopy is the most important step in treating the complication. Additionally, careful dissection will, in most cases, prevent damage to the ureters or colon.

A number of authors have reported side

effects of LPSN related to possible effects of interrupting the presacral nerve, with most of these only lasting two weeks to six months. These include voiding dysfunction, constipation, sexual dysfunction and backache (Malinak, 1980; Rock and Jones, 1983; Lee *et al.*, 1986; Olive and Martin, 1987; Tjaden *et al.*, 1990; Candiani *et al.*, 1992; Perry and Perez, 1993). Urinary complaints have included urge incontinence, urinary incontinence without urgency, difficulty initiating urination, continual leakage of a small amount of urine requiring a sanitary pad and loss of the feeling of a full bladder. Constipation is one of the more common postoperative complaints and is usually easily managed with stool softeners and laxatives. The only form of sexual dysfunction reported is that of occasional vaginal dryness, again usually only temporary. Low back pain, if present, most often disappears after one to three weeks.

DISCUSSION

Laparoscopic presacral neurectomy, performed by a skilled, trained surgeon, is an effective procedure for providing long-term relief for women with midline pelvic pain and dysmenorrhea. Compared to other treatment interventions such as medical treatment with GnRH analogs or LUNA, laparoscopic presacral neurectomy provides more consistent and complete pain relief over long-term follow-up. LPSN, when performed in conjunction with appropriate adjunct procedures such as ablation of endometriosis and lysis of adhesions, is an effective method for an initial surgical treatment of midline dysmenorrhea and pelvic pain.

Only two prospective studies have examined the efficacy of presacral neurectomy in a controlled setting. Tjaden *et al.* (1990) randomly assigned four patients to a presacral neurectomy group and four patients to a non-presacral neurectomy group. Thirteen additional women selected presacral neurectomy for treatment of moderate to severe midline dysmenorrhea and five more selected non-presacral neurectomy treatment alternatives. All 26 subjects completed an 80-item questionnaire prior to surgery and a second questionnaire six months following surgery. The eight patients who were randomly assigned to treatment were not informed of the protocol that they had received until after they completed the six-month follow-up questionnaire. All four of the patients in the presacral neurectomy group reported relief of midline pain at six months, while none of the patients in the non-presacral neurectomy group reported pain relief. Overall results indicated that 15 of the 17 women (88%) who underwent presacral neurectomy experienced pain relief at six months, while none of the nine women who did not have presacral neurectomy experienced pain relief. The study was stopped by the experimental monitoring committee after the first 26 patients were treated, because of concerns about the ethics of depriving future patients of the option of presacral neurectomy for pain relief for midline dysmenorrhea.

Candiani *et al.* (1992) examined the efficacy of presacral neurectomy with adjunct, concurrent procedures to provide relief from pain secondary to moderate to severe endometriosis. Seventy-eight woman were randomly assigned to an experimental group (presacral neurectomy plus conservative surgery) or a control group (conservative surgery only). A multidimensional instrument for measuring the severity of dysmenorrhea and pelvic pain by functional impact on working ability and the need for analgesics and a ten-point linear rating scale to classify pain symptoms (none to severe) were administered to each woman prior to surgery, at six months after surgery and at one year following surgery. One year following surgery, 80% of the patients who were treated with presacral neurectomy and adjunct conservative procedures experienced successful pain relief and 75% of the women who had only conservative surgical procedures had successful pain relief. Candiani and his colleagues concluded that because women with endometriosis often experience lateral pain in addition to midline pain, their study was inconclusive on the increase in effectiveness of presacral neurectomy and adjunct conservative over conservative surgery alone. However, they reinforce the assertion that presacral neurectomy is, in fact, effective for relieving midline pain associated with dysmenorrhea and that while their findings were inconclusive, presacral neurectomy would be indicated in patients with endometriosis and significant midline pain.

It cannot be overemphasized that laparoscopic presacral neurectomy should only be performed by an advanced endoscopic surgeon who has previously demonstrated proficiency in performing presacral neurectomy at laparotomy and who has sufficient skills, at laparotomy and laparoscopy, to manage potential complications such as an accidental laceration of major vessels. The most common side effects of LPSN are transient, but the potential for significant complication from damage to vessels or other structures requires that the surgeon proceed with caution when performing dissection during the laparoscopic presacral neurectomy. The best method for treating a complication is prevention.

Because of the small number of prospective studies and the absence of systematic long-term follow-up in existing retrospective and prospective studies, additional research is needed to show the efficacy of LPSN for long-term pain relief. In addition, further research is indicated to measure the advantages and disadvantages of performing LPSN to relieve midline pain at the same time as adjunct procedures such as ablation of endometriosis and lysis of adhesions for relieving lateral pain.

REFERENCES

Barbot, J. (1989) Hysteroscopy for abnormal bleeding, in *Diagnostic and Operative Hysteroscopy: A Text and Atlas*, (eds. M.S. Baggish, J. Barbot and R.F. Valle), Year Book Medical Publishers, Chicago, pp. 147–55.

Beecham, C.T. (1978) Endometriosis: when is surgical treatment indicated? *PostGrad Med*, **63**, 221–5.

Biggerstaff, E.D. and Foster, S.N. (1994) Laparoscopic presacral neurectomy for the treatment of midline pelvic pain: *J Am Assoc Gynecol Lapar*, **2**, 31–5.

Bird, C.C. and Molitor, J.J. (1971) Adenomyosis: a clinical and pathologic appraisal. *Am J Obstet Gynecol*, **110**, 275–84.

Bird, C.C., McElin, T.W. and Manalo-Estrella, P. (1956) Problems in the diagnosis of adenomyosis uteri, with special reference to dysfunctional bleeding. *West J Surg Obstet Gynecol*, **64**, 291–305.

Bird, C.C., McElin, T.W. and Manalo-Estrella, P. (1972) The elusive adenomyosis of the uterus – revisited. *Am J Obstet Gynecol*, **112**, 583–93.

Black, W.T. (1964) Use of presacral sympathectomy in the treatment of dysmenorrhea. *Am J Obstet Gynecol*, **89**, 16–22.

Bonica, J.J. (1975) The nature of pain in parturition. *Clin Obstet Gynecol*, **2**, 499.

Bonica, J.J. (ed.) (1990) *The Management of Pain*, 2nd edn, Lea and Febinger, Philadelphia.

Candiani, G.B., Fedele, L., Vercellini, P. *et al.* (1992) Presacral neurectomy for the treatment of pelvic pain associated with endometriosis: a controlled study. *Am J Obstet Gynecol*, **167**, 100–103.

Cleland, J.G.P. (1933) Paravertebral anesthesia in obstetrics. *Surg Gynecol Obstet*, **57**, 51.

Clemente, C.D. (ed.) (1985) *Gray's Anatomy of the Human Body*, 30th edn, Lea and Febinger, Philadelphia.

Cotte, G. (1937) Resection of the presacral nerve in the treatment of obstinate dysmenorrhea. *Am J Obstet Gynecol*, **33**, 1034–40.

Counsellor, V.S. and Craig, M.W. (1934) The treatment of dysmenorrhea by resection of the presacral sympathetic nerves: evaluation of end-results. *Am J Obstet Gynecol*, **28**, 161–72.

Courtois, C.A. (1988) *Healing the Incest Wound: Adult Survivors in Therapy*, W.W. Norton, New York.

Cullen, T.S. (1908) *Adenomyoma of Uterus*, W.B. Saunders, Philadelphia.

Daniell, J.F., Kurtz, B.R., Gurley, L. and Lalonde, C. (1993) Laparoscopic presacral neurectomy vs neurotomy: use of the argon beam coagulator compared to conventional technique. *J Gynecol Surg*, **9**, 169–73.

Davis, A.A. (1933) The technique of resection of the presacral nerve (Cotte's operation). *Br J Surg*, **20**, 516–20.

Doyle, J.B. (1955) Paracervical uterine denervation by transection of the cervical plexus for the relief of dysmenorrhea. *Am J Obstet Gynecol*, **70**, 1–16.

Elaut, L. (1933) The surgical anatomy of the so-called presacral nerve. *Surg Gynecol Obstet*, **57**, 581–9.

Evans, T.N. (1971) Office gynecological problems, in *Textbook of Obstetrics and Gynecology*, (ed. D.N. Danforth), Harper and Row, Hagerstown, MD.

Fedele, L., Arcaini, L., Bianchi, S. *et al.* (1989) Comparison of cyproterone acetate and danazol in the treatment of pelvic pain associated with endometriosis. *Obstet Gynecol*, **73**, 1000–1005.

Fedele, L., Bianchi, S., Boccidone, L. *et al.* (1993) Buserelin acetate in the treatment of pelvic pain associated with minimal and mild endometriosis: a controlled study. *Fertil Steril*, **59**, 516–21.

Fliegner, J.R.H. and Umstad, M.P. (1991) Presacral neurectomy – a reappraisal. *Aust NZ J Obstet Gynaecol*, **31**, 76–9.

Fontaine, R. and Herrmann, L.G. (1932) Clinical and experimental basis for surgery of the pelvic sympathetic nerves in gynecology. *Surg Gynecol Obstet*, **54**, 133–63.

Greenblatt, R.B., Dmowski, W.P. *et al.* (1971) Clinical studies with an anti-gonadotropin – Danazol. *Fertil Steril*, **22**, 102–112.

Greenhill, J.P. (1965) *Obstetrics*, 13th edn., W.B. Saunders, Philadelphia.

Gürgan, T., Urman, B. *et al.* (1992) Laparoscopic CO_2 laser uterine nerve ablation for treatment of drug resistant primary dysmenorrhea. *Fertil Steril*, **58**, 422–24.

Head, H. (1893) On disturbances of sensation with special reference to the pain of visceral disease. *Brain*, **16**, 1.

Herman, J.L. (1992) *Trauma and Recovery*, Pandora, London.

Hill, D.J. and Maher, P.J. (1991) Letter to the editor. *Aust NZ J Obstet Gynaecol*, **31**, 290.

Kistner, R.W. (1979) Endometriosis and infertility. *Clin Obstet Gynecol*, **22**, 101–119.

Lee, R.B., Stone, K. *et al.* (1986) Presacral neurectomy for chronic pelvic pain. *Obstet Gynecol*, **68**, 517–521.

Lichten, E.M. and Bombard, J. (1987) Surgical treatment of dysmenorrhea with laparoscopic uterine nerve ablation. *J Reprod Med*, **32**, 37–41.

Mahfoud, H.K. and Hewitt, S.R. (1981) A place for presacral neurectomy. *Irish Med J*, **74**, 198–199.

Malinak, L.R. (1980) Operative management of pelvic pain. *Clin Obstet Gynecol*, **23**, 191–200.

Martin, D.C., Hubert, G.D. *et al.* (1989) Laparoscopic appearance of peritoneal endometriosis. *Fertil Steril*, **51**, 63–67.

McCoy, J.B. and Bradford, W.Z. (1963) Surgical treatment of endometriosis and conservation of reproductive potential. *Am J Obstet Gynecol*, **87**, 394–398.

Meldrum, D.R., Chang, R.J., Lu, J. *et al.* (1987) 'Medical oophorectomy' using a long-acting GnRH agonist: a possible new approach to the treatment of endometriosis. *J Clin Endocrinol Metab*, **54**, 1081–3.

Namnoum, A.B., Hickman, T. N., Goodman, S. *et al.* (1993) *Incidence of Symptom Recurrence Following Hysterectomy for Endometriosis*. Paper presented at the Conjoint Meeting of the American Fertility Society and the Canadian Fertility and Andrology Society, October 11–14, Montreal.

Nishida, M. (1991) Relationship between the onset of dysmenorrhea and histological findings in adenomyosis. *Am J Obstet Gynecol*, **165**, 229–31.

Nezhat, C. and Nezhat, F. (1992) A simplified method of laparoscopic presacral neurectomy for the treatment of central pelvic pain due to endometriosis. *Br J Obstet Gynaecol*, **99**, 659–63.

Olive, D.L. and Martin, D.C. (1987) Treatment of endometriosis-associated infertility with CO_2 laparoscopy: the use of one and two parameter exponential models. *Fertil Steril*, **48**, 18–23.

Pastner, B. and Orr, J.W. (1990) Intractable venous sacral hemorrhage: use of stainless steel thumbtacks to obtain hemostasis. *Am J Obstet Gynecol*, **162**, 452.

Perez, J.J. (1990) Laparoscopic presacral neurectomy: results of the first 25 cases. *J Reprod Med*, **35**, 625–30.

Perry, C.P. and Perez, J. (1993) The role for laparoscopic presacral neurectomy. *J Gynecol Surg*, **9**, 165–8.

Peterson, H.B., Hulka, J.F., Phillips, J. *et al.* (1990) American Association of Gynecologic Laparoscopists 1988 membership survey on operative laparoscopy. *J Reprod Med*, **35**, 587–9.

Polan, M.L. and DeCherney, A. (1980) Presacral neurectomy for pelvic pain in infertility. *Fertil Steril*, **34**, 557–60.

Pritchard, J.A., McDonald, P.C. and Gant, N.F. (eds) (1985) *Williams Obstetrics*, 17th edn, Appleton-Century-Crofts, Norwalk, CT.

Renaer, M. and Guzinski, G.M. (1978) Pain in gynecologic practice. *Pain*, **5**, 305–31.

Rock, J. and Jones, H. (1983) Endometriosis externa, in *Reparative and Constructive Surgery of the Female Generative Tract*, (ed. H.W. Jones), Williams and Wilkins, Baltimore, pp. 136–8.

Sackier, J.M. (1993) Visualization of the ureter during laparoscopic colonic resection. *Br J Surg*, **80**, 1332.

Seibel, R.M.M. and Gronemeyer, D.H.W. (1990) CT-guided neurolysis of the presacral and precoccygeal sympathetic trunk, in *Interventional Computed Tomography*, (eds R.M. Seibel and D.H.W. Gronemeyer), Blackwell Scientific, Boston.

Steingold, K.A., Cedars, L., Lu, J. *et al.* (1987) Treatment of endometriosis with a long-acting gonadotropin-releasing hormone agonist. *Obstet Gynecol*, **69**, 403–11.

Sutton, C.J.G. (1992) What can we expect from the surgical management of endometriosis? *Br J Clin Pract*, **72**(suppl), 33–44.

Tjaden, B., Schlaff, W.D., Kimball, A. *et al.* (1990) The efficacy of presacral neurectomy for the relief of midline dysmenorrhea. *Obstet Gynecol*, **76**, 89–91.

Walker, E., Katon, W., Harrops-Griffuths, J. *et al.* (1988) Relationship of chronic pelvic pain to psychiatric diagnoses and childhood sexual abuse. *Am J Psychiatry*, **145**, 75–80.

Wharton, L.R. (1977) Presacral neurectomy, in *TeLinda's Operative Gynecology*, 5th edn (ed. R.E. Mattingly), J.P. Lippincott, Philadelphia, p. 254.

Williams, P.L. and Warwick, R. (eds.) (1980) *Gray's Anatomy*, 36th edn, W.B. Saunders, Philadelphia.

LAPAROSCOPIC AND ULTRASOUND-GUIDED TRANSVAGINAL MANAGEMENT AND IMAGING OF BENIGN OVARIAN TUMORS

S. Ewen, W. Walker and C.J.G. Sutton

INTRODUCTION

The majority of gynecological operations can now be performed by laparoscopic surgical techniques and this is particularly true of the management of benign ovarian tumors. The real problem facing the gynecologist is to be as certain as humanly possible that the tumor is benign before surgery commences.

All adnexal masses should be carefully screened by vaginal ultrasound imaging, regardless of the age of the patient. They should be less than 10 cm in diameter with distinct borders and have no evidence of irregular solid parts, thick or numerous septae, ascites or matted bowel and postmenopausal patients should not have an elevated CA125 level. With the increasing sophistication of imaging techniques it should be possible to be almost completely certain of the pathological diagnosis before operation, but the laparoscopic surgeon must always be vigilant in cases of unsuspected carcinoma or borderline malignancy for tissue retrieval, as early stage disease has been successfully treated by minimal access surgery.

It is not necessary to treat all cysts laparoscopically. At our institution we have been treating a selected group of benign simple cysts by ultrasound-guided cyst aspiration since the early 1980s.

PREOPERATIVE DIAGNOSIS AND IMAGING

The improvement in ultrasound technology, particularly the introduction of high frequency transvaginal scanners, has considerably facilitated the assessment of ovarian cysts and in particular visualization of their internal architecture. Numerous publications have assessed the ability of ultrasound to distinguish benign from malignant lesions, some indicating a high degree of success (Meire *et al.*, 1978; Herrmann *et al.*, 1987) and others showing a lower correlation (Granberg *et al.*, 1990). Generally speaking, cysts containing papillary projections, solid areas, thick septae or outer walls have a higher incidence of malignancy. Solid areas are particularly suspicious (Granberg *et al.*, 1989a, 1990).

UNILOCULAR CYSTS

Unlike complex cysts, in the case of unilocular thinwalled ovarian cysts ultrasound carries a high positive predictive value for benign disease (Meire *et al.*, 1978; Deland *et al.*, 1979; Moyle *et al.*, 1983; Granberg *et al.*, 1989a, 1990). Thus ultrasound-guided cyst aspiration has been used as a method for diagnosis and treatment of such cysts (de Crespigny, 1985; Granberg *et al.*, 1989b; Kaw and Walker, 1990; Bret *et al.*, 1992a).

Gynecological Endoscopic Surgery. Edited by C.J.G. Sutton. Published in 1997 by Chapman & Hall, London.
ISBN 0 412 58040 3.

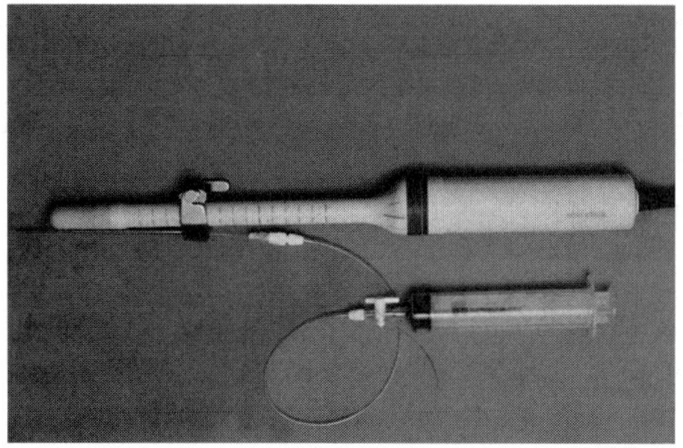

Figure 7.1   Transvaginal probe for the technique of aspiration.

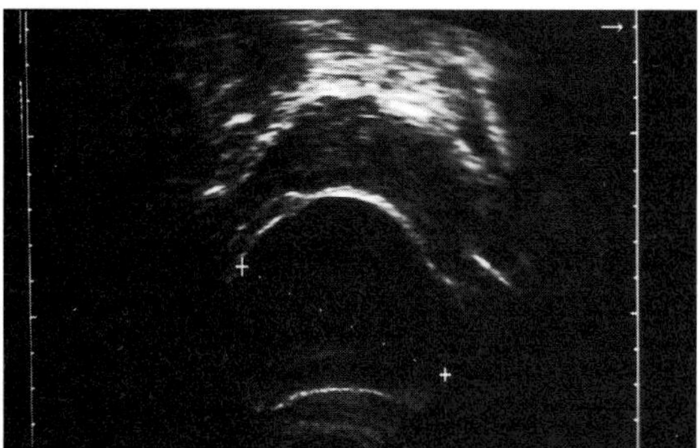

Figure 7.2   Transvaginal scan of pelvis showing typical unilocular cyst in pouch of Douglas.

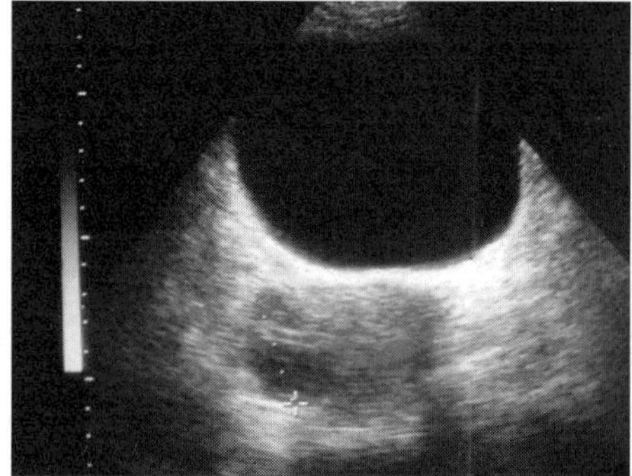

(a)

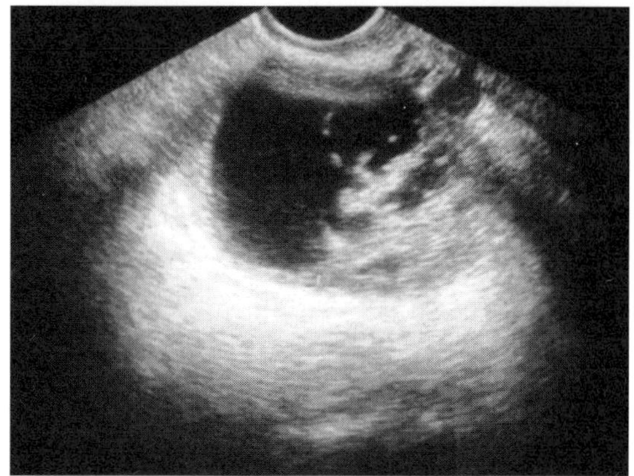

(b)

Figure 7.3   (a) Transabdominal scan showing right ovarian abnormality inadequately defined. (b) Transvaginal scan of same case demonstrating cystic ovarian carcinoma with solid component penetrating through ovarian capsule.

Cyst aspiration can be performed either transabdominally, usually through the bladder, or using transabdominal scanning but puncturing through the vagina via a speculum or lastly through the vaginal fornix using a transvaginal scanner (Figure 7.1). The latter is the most efficacious and most aspirations are carried out in this way. It is essential that prior to evacuating the cyst a very careful ultrasound examination is performed by a skilled operator to insure that the cyst is truly unilocular and thinwalled (a few thin septae are usually acceptable) (Figure 7.2).

It is not difficult to miss small papillary excrescences or slight thickenings of the wall in unilocular cysts by either transabdominal or transvaginal scanning. In a small number of cases transvaginal scanning may not reveal detail of the base of a cyst because of its proximity to the probe, or in very large cysts part of the wall may be beyond the range of the transducer; in such difficult cases transabdominal scanning is also necessary. Transabdominal scanning alone, however, is insufficient for assessment prior to cyst aspiration as in a proportion of cases there is simply inadequate resolution of the internal architecture (Figure 7.3).

ULTRASOUND-GUIDED TRANSVAGINAL CYST ASPIRATION

This is normally carried out using a fine gauge needle (20–22 gauge), but if the fluid is viscous then larger needles (16–18 gauge) are necessary, particularly for draining endometriotic cysts. Anesthesia and sedation are usually unnecessary for cyst puncture and most workers do not administer antibiotic cover prior to the procedure. To our knowledge only one infective complication has been reported in the literature (Zanetta *et al.*, 1993). However, our group has recorded one ovarian abscess from a large series of transvaginal aspirations and antibiotic cover is therefore given routinely. The cyst is usually aspirated to dryness and some workers flush the cyst with saline and reaspirate, theoretically in order to increase the retrieval of cells from the cyst wall for cytology. However, this has not been shown to be effective (Granberg *et al.*, 1989b). Follow-up by repeat ultrasound examinations is then necessary to insure that the cyst has resolved.

Most unilocular cysts in premenopausal women will be of the follicular type, some will be corpus luteum cysts and others true simple cysts. Many unilocular cysts resolve without aspiration, but often patients are symptomatic and aspiration of these cysts removes symptoms and probably speeds resolution. It might be argued that the cysts that resolve (approximately 50–70% following aspiration) are those that would probably resolve spontaneously at some time in the future in any case, but as yet this is unknown.

HEMORRHAGIC CYSTS

Hemorrhagic cysts are a special case; they are often heterogeneous, of varying echogenicity and may even appear to have numerous locules. However, they usually occur in patients with a typical history. Most are functional cysts with hemorrhage and many will resolve spontaneously (Baltarowich *et al.*, 1987). Aspiration reveals recently blood-stained fluid and usually induces resolution of symptoms. In our series of 17 hemorrhagic, non-endometriotic ovarian cysts, 71% resolved after cyst aspiration. Some workers have attempted sclerosis of ovarian cysts with

the introduction of transvaginal alcohol (Bret *et al.*, 1992b) but the role of this procedure is probably limited (Thurmond, 1992).

EXCLUSION OF MALIGNANCY

The crucial question with regard to the conservative management of unilocular cysts (i.e. observation) versus transvaginal cyst aspiration is whether there is a likelihood that a malignant cyst may be missed despite ultrasound assessment and cytology of the aspirated fluid. We know that cystadenomas, both mucinous and serous, may be entirely unilocular and anechoic. Such cysts need to be diagnosed and removed as malignant transformation may be a possibility. Evidence for the latter mainly relies on the coexistence of benign and malignant epithelium in the walls of malignant cyst adenocarcinomas. Unfortunately cytology of the aspirated fluid cannot be relied on to differentiate between benign borderline and frankly malignant cysts (Diernaes *et al.*, 1987; Kaw and Walker, 1990; Granberg *et al.*, 1991; Dordoni *et al.*, 1993; Granberg and Wikland, 1993). It may be that assessment of the levels of CEA and CA125 in the aspirated fluid would be useful (Pinto *et al.*, 1990).

Color Doppler examination of ovarian cysts was greeted with considerable initial enthusiasm but more recent reports appear to show an inadequate positive predictive value (Bourne, 1991; Weiner *et al.*, 1993). However, combined with CA125 estimation and assessment of the internal architecture of cysts it is probably a useful tool (Kurjak and Predanic, 1992).

Assessment of serum CA125 appears to be useful, particularly as an adjunct to ultrasonic assessment of ovarian cysts (Finkler *et al.*, 1988). However, CA125 may not pick up the well-differentiated adenocarcinoma or cysts of borderline malignancy. The efficacy of CA125 estimation in unilocular ovarian cysts which are malignant or of borderline malignancy is unknown. In addition, CA125 levels can be elevated (often considerably) in cases of endometriosis and many other conditions which can cause confusion in premenopausal women.

Cyst aspiration or conservative treatment of unilocular cysts is based on the fact that the incidence of malignancy in unilocular cysts is extremely low. Granberg and Wikland (1991) quote an incidence of 0.3%. Other authors (Meire *et al.*, 1978; Deland *et al.*, 1979; Moyle *et al.*, 1993) give higher incidences in the order of 4–5%. However, the ultrasonic criteria are slightly different. In our experience of cyst aspiration in 126 pregnant and non-pregnant patients the incidence of borderline or malignant unilocular cysts was less then 1%. Much, however, will depend on the experience and accuracy of the ultrasonographer in assessing the cysts and it is important that subtle changes in cyst morphology are appreciated. It could be argued that a positive predictive value even of 95% is inadequate to justify conservative therapy. However, this has to be set against the complications of diagnostic laparoscopy which are significant (Mintz, 1977; Parewijck *et al.*, 1979; Kane and Krejs, 1984; Peterson *et al.*, 1990), compared with the negligible complications of ultrasound-guided aspiration published so far (Zanetta *et al.*, 1993). It is mandatory that if cysts recur after one or two aspirations they should be submitted to laparoscopy and removed as a significant majority will turn out to be cyst adenomas.

MANAGEMENT OF OVARIAN CYSTS IN POSTMENOPAUSAL WOMEN

The role of conservative therapy and transvaginal cyst aspiration in postmenopausal women with cysts is still unclear. It certainly appears that most cysts in postmenopausal women are benign (Herrmann *et al.*, 1987; Goldstein and Subramanyam, 1989). It would seem, therefore, that there is a rationale for treating the cysts conservatively, as advocated by Andolf and Jorgensen (1988), or by

transvaginal aspiration. The recurrence rate, however, of postmenopausal cysts is greater than in premenopausal women (Dordoni *et al.*, 1993) due to the lack of functional cysts and more will be cyst adenomas or cyst adenofibromas. In general small unilocular ovarian cysts in postmenopausal patients under 5 cm in size may be either monitored regularly or aspirated. If the cysts are over 5 cm transvaginal aspiration may be attempted but if the cyst recurs it should be removed by laparoscopic surgery.

MANAGEMENT OF OVARIAN CYSTS IN PREGNANCY

Only one article in the world literature has included a series of ultrasound-guided cyst aspirations in pregnancy (Figure 7.4) (Kaw and Walker, 1990).

The prevalence of cysts in the first half of pregnancy is 1 in 190 and the incidence of malignant cysts approximately 1 in 127 (Hogston and Lilford, 1986). Torsion of cysts is more common in pregnancy (Dewhurst, 1981), with a 29% incidence of torsion in *symptomatic* cysts of which almost half are functional (Buttery *et al.*, 1973). Dewhurst (1981) and Myerscough (1982) advocated the removal of all cysts in the second trimester. However,

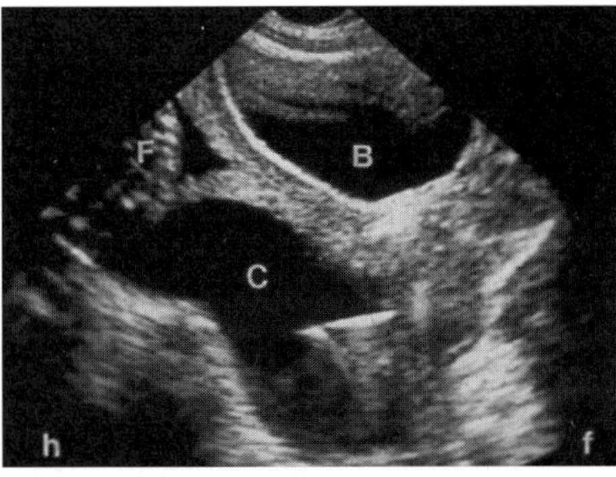

Figure 7.4 Transabdominal scan during pregnancy showing needle inserted through vaginal fornix into large benign cyst. B = bladder, C = cyst, F = fetus.

Hogston and Lilford (1986) demonstrated that most cysts in pregnancy are functional and will resolve and may be treated conservatively depending on their ultrasonic characteristics. Certainly surgery in pregnancy carries a risk to both mother and fetus and a fetal loss rate from surgery of 26% (Hill *et al.*, 1975). Transvaginal aspiration of cysts may therefore reduce the risk of torsion, rupture or obstruction of labor or complications from surgery. If reaccumulation of the cyst occurs the procedure can easily be repeated (Kaw and Walker, 1990).

FINE NEEDLE ASPIRATION OF COMPLEX CYSTS AND SOLID TUMORS

Finally, fine needle aspiration of complex ovarian cysts or solid ovarian tumors may be useful in that if the cytological evaluation is positive for malignancy, this helps the surgeon plan the operation. Cytology is likely to be positive in the case of poorly differentiated tumors and those with marked papillary proliferation. A contraindication to the puncture of malignant cysts was thought to be the possibility of disseminated malignant cells along the needle track. This, however, appears unlikely (Livraghi *et al.*, 1983). Where cytology is positive fine needle aspiration biopsy of malignant lesions is useful to the surgeon in planning the approach to surgery.

The one situation where needling of a cyst may be contraindicated is if there is a reasonable suspicion of a teratoma (dermoid). In this situation leakage of the sebaceous material can induce a chemical peritonitis, resulting in severe abdominal pain (Zanetta *et al.*, 1993).

LAPAROSCOPIC ASSESSMENT OF AN OVARIAN NEOPLASM

Assuming that there are no ultrasonic features suggestive of malignancy and any cyst fluid aspirated by fine needle aspiration is negative for malignant cells, it is safe to proceed to laparoscopy. Nevertheless, patients should be aware that ultrasonic diagnosis is not 100% reliable and should be warned that if features suspicious of malignancy are found at laparoscopy the correct course of action is to proceed to laparotomy and they should have consented to this (Nezhat *et al.*, 1991). Having said that, it must be realized that many modern women would object to removal of their ovaries without a full and frank discussion and a body of opinion would suggest full laparoscopic staging and review of histology and then laparotomy after discussion with the patient.

All visible peritoneal surfaces, including the dome of the diaphragm, the liver, the digestive tract and the omentum, should be carefully inspected for metastases. Any fluid in the pouch of Douglas is aspirated for cytological examination and then the peritoneal surface of the pelvis and lower abdomen are irrigated with heparinized Hartman's solution and the resulting washings aspirated for cytological examination. The ovarian surface of both ovaries must be carefully scrutinized under magnification for external papillary projections and, if present, these and any suspicious peritoneal appearances should be biopsied and sent for frozen section. If adhesions are present, a gentle adhesiolysis may first have to be performed with laser or scissors. The utero-ovarian ligament should be observed and lengthening of this ligament is often an indirect sign of a non-functional cyst (Audebert, 1993).

The ovaries are gently grasped with forceps, usually at the insertion of the ovarian ligament, but great care must be taken to avoid tearing the ovary at this site because it can be extremely vascular. If internal papillary projections have not been visualized on ultrasound examination a needle can be used to aspirate the fluid content, taking care to avoid unnecessary spillage. It is possible to perform ovarioscopy with a fine endoscope in much the same way as salpingoscopy is performed (Brosens and Puttemans, 1989). If such equipment is not available it is possible to enlarge the puncture site with scissors and carefully inspect the inside of the cyst wall with the magnification afforded by the 10 mm laparoscope held close against the internal surface of the cyst. Any suspicious areas should be biopsied and sent for frozen section if this facility is available. If at any stage of this assessment there is the remotest suspicion of malignancy or a teratoma (see below) it is safer to perform these maneuvers within a plastic retrieval bag to avoid the possibility of spillage of potentially malignant tissue (Adelson, 1991).

LAPAROSCOPIC OVARIAN CYSTECTOMY

Most benign ovarian cysts can be treated laparoscopically, either by stripping the cyst capsule after fenestration (Figure 7.5) or by removing the ovarian cyst intact. In younger patients an attempt should be made to conserve as much of the ovarian tissue as possible. The CO_2 laser can be used to establish a plane of cleavage between the cyst wall and the ovarian cortex and, if a laser is not available, this can be performed with a microdiathermy needle. It is important to make the incision relatively superficial to avoid puncturing the

cyst, especially in the case of a dermoid, and this tissue plane can be further developed by aquadissection or instrument traction and countertraction by the strong grasp of two pairs of ovarian biopsy forceps until the cyst is removed *in toto*. Caution is constantly exercised to avoid puncture of the cyst wall and spillage of the contents, but the risk of disseminating any tumor cells if malignancy has been missed in the preoperative work-up is more theoretical than real (Dembo *et al.*, 1990; Sevelda *et al.*, 1990; Finn *et al.*, 1992).

The most difficult part of the operation is the removal of the ovarian cyst, particularly if it is larger than 5 cm or if it is a dermoid containing material that could irritate the peritoneum if inadvertently spilled. It can usually be removed through an enlarged umbilical incision by pulling it out at the same time as the 10 mm trocar, grasping its edges with hemostats and, if necessary, decompressing it by aspirating the contents through the umbilical incision.

If the ovary has to be removed intact, a posterior colpotomy incision is made with the laser or microdiathermy needle between the uterosacral ligaments, using as a backstop a moist gauze swab in the posterior vaginal

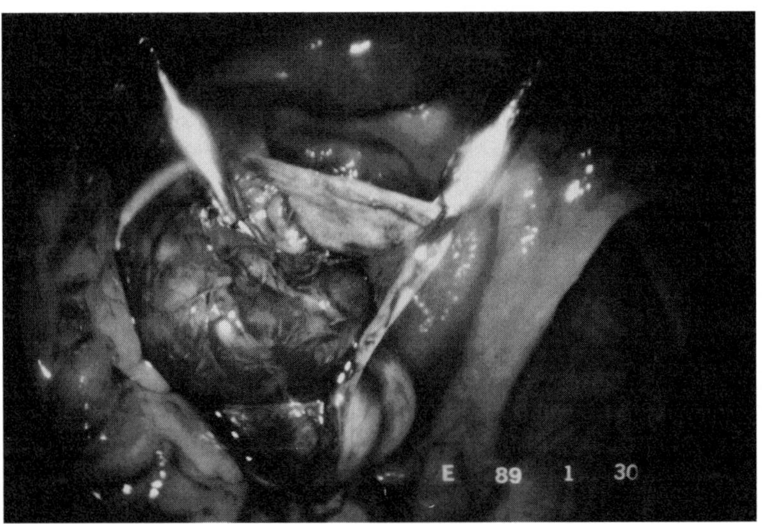

Figure 7.5 Laparoscopic ovarian cystectomy by stripping the cyst lining.

Table 7.1 Evaluation of 652 women with ovarian tumors (Mage *et al.*, 1990)

Laparoscopy	N	Func	Benign	LMP	Cancer
			Pathologic diagnosis		
Functional	109	96	13	0	0
Benign	517	15	502	0	0
Suspicious	21	0	14	5	2
Cancer	5	0	0	1	4
Total	652	111	529	6	6

fornix to identify the incision site and to absorb laser energy (Davis and Herubi, 1989). If the ovarian cyst is removed through a colpotomy incision it is essential to warn the pathologist, otherwise the ovarian surface will be contaminated with vaginal squames, making histological interpretation very difficult. If there is any concern about borderline malignancy or if the cyst is a dermoid, then it should be removed within a retrieval bag which is most easily removed through a posterior colpotomy incision.

RESULTS OF LAPAROSCOPIC TREATMENT
OF OVARIAN TUMORS

The largest published series of ovarian cysts managed by laparoscopy is from Clermont-Ferrand in France (Mage *et al.*, 1990; Canis *et al.*, 1994) and this includes 652 ovarian cysts of which six were ovarian cancers and six borderline malignant neoplasms (Table 7.1). All of these were identified at the time of diagnostic laparoscopy and treated immediately by laparotomy. Audebert (1993) has evaluated 308 women (some with bilateral lesions) and found eight malignant or borderline neoplasms, all of which were managed by laparotomy except one which was managed by laparoscopy. She was a woman of 35 and has been carefully checked and followed up and the second ovary was removed three years later but no evidence of malignancy was detected.

At this moment in time metastatic ovarian malignancy is best managed by primary debulking at laparotomy (Mage *et al.*, 1990; Gleeson *et al.*, 1993), but there have been individual cases of stage I disease being treated laparoscopically (Reich *et al.*, 1990) and with the increasing use of retrieval bags together with pelvic and para-aortic node sampling performed by laparoscopy, this may in fact be the treatment of choice for early ovarian malignancy in the future. The role of laparoscopic surgery in gynecologic oncology has been extensively reviewed in an article by Michel Canis (Canis *et al.*, 1994) in the light of the extensive experience of Professor Bruhat's team from Clermont-Ferrand, France, but will need to be carefully evaluated before it can be universally recommended.

LAPAROSCOPIC TREATMENT OF TUBO-OVARIAN ABSCESS

Pelvic infection is very poorly treated in current gynecological practice, with reliance placed on aggressive antibiotic therapy which often seems to result in dense and extensive adhesions involving bowel, pelvic peritoneum and omentum and ending with the distressing symptoms of chronic pelvic pain and infertility. Laparoscopic intervention offers an opportunity to prevent these long-term sequelae (Reich and McGlynn, 1987; Johns, 1993).

Intravenous antibiotics are given to rapidly establish an adequate blood level before embarking on laparoscopic aquadissection, whereby the entire abdominal cavity is rinsed with warm Ringer's lactate solution under pressure to gently break down the filmy adhesions, open up the abscess cavity and remove all the pus, blood and debris. This laparoscopic procedure requires a minimum of equipment, merely a blunt probe and aquadissector, but a maximum amount of patience on the part of the surgeon. The inflammatory exudate lining the abscess cavity and all the necrotic debris covering the pelvic organs are removed by gentle teasing with ovarian biopsy forceps and aquadissection. At the end of the procedure 1–2 liters of warm irrigant fluid is left in the abdominal cavity to dilute any remaining bacteria and to 'aquafloat' the pelvic contents to decrease the possibility of adhesion formation, which usually occurs during the first four postoperative hours (MacDonald and Sutton, 1992). Following this revolutionary approach to pelvic sepsis, the patients recover rapidly and second-look laparoscopy reveals a remarkably normal-looking pelvis, any filmy adhesions simply being lyzed by the carbon dioxide laser or scissor dissection.

LAPAROSCOPIC REMOVAL OF TERATOMAS (DERMOIDS)

Benign ovarian teratomas, otherwise known as dermoid cysts, tend to occur in the younger age group and account for 10–15% of all ovarian tumors. Malignant teratomas are rare but do occur in 1–3% of cases. Before the advent of minimally invasive surgery the standard management for dermoid cysts was laparotomy and ovarian cystectomy or oophorectomy. The cysts can, however, be removed laparoscopically but clearly the main problem they present is the risk of rupture and spillage of the thick sebaceous material which may also include hair, teeth or other solid components and can induce a severe chemical peritonitis.

There are three main approaches to the laparoscopic removal of these cysts. Firstly, a small opening can be made through the cyst wall with laser, needle point diathermy or scissors and then the cyst contents aspirated and the cyst flushed. The aim is to keep spillage to a minimum to avoid peritoneal irritation, but this procedure can be difficult due to the thick contents of the dermoid. Once the cyst contents have been aspirated the cyst lining is freed from the surrounding ovarian tissue and then removed through one of the abdominal trocars. The abdomen is repeatedly irrigated to remove all debris.

In order to prevent spillage of cyst contents into the abdominal cavity, the cyst aspiration can be carried out within a retrieval bag. The Endocatch (Autosuture, Ascot, UK) has two metal springs to open the bag but some retrieval bags without this mechanism can be surprisingly difficult to open. A simple practical tip is to expand the bag with a jet of fluid from the irrigator which expands the bag uniformly and allows early insertion of the cyst follicle by suction of the remaining fluid. Technically, the most delicate stage of the operation is extraction of the cyst and this technique is particularly complicated if the cyst is large or has an important solid component. This problem can be overcome by performing a laparoscopic ovarian cystectomy into a bag and then removing the cyst and cyst contents in the bag via a posterior colpotomy. A third approach has recently been reported (Dubuisson and Chapron, 1994), which involves exteriorizing the dermoid cyst through a minilaparotomy incision to effect its removal. If there is no normal ovarian tissue to be found separate from the dermoid cyst then clearly an oophorectomy can be performed laparoscopically.

LAPAROSCOPIC TREATMENT OF OVARIAN ENDOMETRIOMAS

Ovarian endometriomas are invariably unresponsive to drug therapy and whilst some shrinkage occurs after several months of treatment with luteinizing hormone-releasing analogs, they almost invariably regrow when therapy is discontinued (Donnez *et al.*, 1992).

With advances in minimally invasive surgery it is now possible to treat large endometriomas and severe endometriosis by the laparoscopic approach (Sutton, 1993). Some surgeons employ a three-stage technique with initial drainage of the cyst, interval therapy with LHRH analogs for three months followed by laparoscopic surgery with dissection and removal of the cyst lining (Bruhat *et al.*, 1989) or CO_2 laser vaporization of the cyst lining (Donnez *et al.*, 1989). The KTP/532 flexible fiber laser is a very effective tool for the

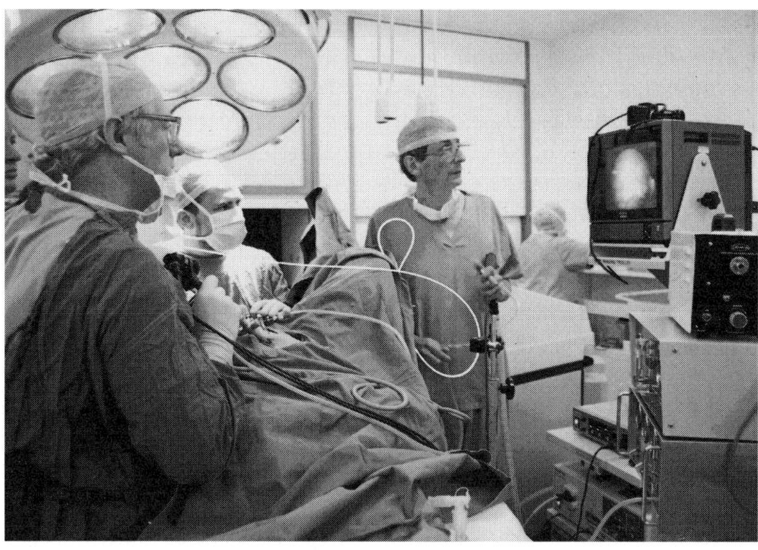

Figure 7.6   KTP laser photocoagulation of endometrioma.

photocoagulation of the endometriotic cyst lining (Daniell *et al.*, 1991; Marrs, 1991), and this has also been our experience (Figure 7.6, Plate 2).

We have recently reviewed a series of 102 patients with endometriomas ranging in size from 3 to 18 cm with pain, infertility or both. The mean AFS score was 45 and the mean duration of infertility was for 53 months. Most of the patients were tertiary referrals and had undergone numerous previous treatments, including several attempts at assisted conception (Sutton, 1995). Sixty-six out of 84 patients (78%) reported improvement or resolution of their pain and 24 out of 42 infertile patients (57%) achieved a pregnancy.

Although some authors have advocated ovarian closure with laparoscopic sutures, this is illogical since the ischemia produced by surgical knots is associated with an increased likelihood of postoperative adhesion formation (Buckman *et al.*, 1976). Fayez and Vogel (1991) in a prospective study compared four different methods of laparoscopic treatment of endometriomas – wedge incision, stripping of the lining, CO_2 laser vaporization of the lining

and drainage alone. All patients were given danazol for eight weeks and a second-look laparoscopy was performed during the last week of treatment. Although there was no significant difference in the recurrence rate, the excision group all had periadnexal adhesions whereas there was only about a 30% incidence in the other group. For these reasons the authors advised against excision and found the other methods equally efficacious, although this was not a study on infertile patients. Furthermore, formal dissection of an endometrioma that is densely adherent to the ovarian tissue can take a considerable length of time whereas simple incision, drainage and photocoagulation of the endometrioma by laser is a much shorter procedure associated with equivalent or somewhat better results (Sutton, 1995).

LAPAROSCOPIC MANAGEMENT OF ACUTE ADNEXAL TORSION

Adnexal torsion is a rare cause of acute pelvic pain and most frequently occurs if there is an adnexal lesion present. Traditional management has been by laparotomy with excision of the torted ovary without untwisting the pedicle to avoid the risk of embolization from the occluded ovarian veins (Way, 1946; Hibbard, 1985). However, there have been an increasing number of reports recently suggesting that a more conservative approach can be undertaken (Manhes *et al.*, 1992). Zweizig *et al.* (1993) report a retrospective review of 94 women who had undergone surgery for torsion and they concluded that untwisting of the adnexae and ovarian cystectomy can be performed in reproductive age women with adnexal torsion in the absence of a grossly necrotic adnexa. Intravenous fluorescein injection intraoperatively to detect viable fallopian and ovarian tissues involved in adnexal torsion has also been reported and may be a useful adjunct in the conservative management of adnexal torsion. Laparoscopic management of the torted cyst can be achieved by either oophorectomy, if the ovary appears unviable after untwisting, or alternatively untwisting with aspiration or excision of the cyst. This has been reported by Harry Reich (Reich *et al.*, 1992) without any serious sequelae.

LAPAROSCOPIC TREATMENT OF POLYCYSTIC OVARIAN SYNDROME

Polycystic ovarian syndrome (PCOS) is the most common cause of anovulation and it is well accepted that the first approach to ovulation induction in these patients is with the administration of clomiphene citrate. Between 15% and 20% will remain anovulatory and, furthermore, there is a discrepancy between the ovulation rate and the conception rate in these women. Further medical therapy does exist to treat women who are resistant to clomiphene citrate, utilizing either human menopausal gonadotropins or follicle-stimulating hormone. However, in recent years, there has been a swing back towards surgery. Ovarian wedge resection is well known to produce ovulation rates in the region of 80–90%. However, there is an unacceptably high rate of

adhesion formation causing future problems with fertility (Toaff *et al.*, 1976).

Laparoscopic ovarian drilling with cautery was first described by Gjonnaess in 1984 and since then there have been a number of reports of drilling of polycystic ovaries utilizing either electrocoagulation or laser. Naether *et al.* (1993) reported on 133 patients with polycystic ovarian disease and infertility who underwent laparoscopic electrocoagulation of the ovarian surface with a resultant pregnancy rate of 70%. Similarly, Amar and Lachelin (1993), using ovarian diathermy at laparoscopy, reported an 86% ovulation response. Overall, most reports suggest ovulation between 70% and 90% following these procedures, with pregnancy rates between 60% and 80%. A degree of caution, however, needs to be exercised in recommending these procedures before traditional therapy has been exhausted because there is a risk of adhesion formation.

Greenblatt (1993) recently reported early results of a randomized blinded prospective study to evaluate the incidence of postoperative adhesion formation following laparoscopic ovarian cautery and its potential prevention with the use of Interceed. At the time of ovarian cautery, Interceed was placed over the surface of one ovary selected at random and all patients underwent a second-look laparoscopy 3–6 weeks later by a second surgeon who was unaware which ovary had been treated. Total adhesion score at the time of second-look procedure ranged from 2 (minimal) to 42 (severe). There was no consistent correlation between the adhesion score and the site where the Interceed had been applied. All of the patients had some degree of ovarian adhesions. He also concluded that there is a risk of postoperative adhesion formation and until more complete, long-term information is known, caution must be exercised and complete information provided to the patient with respect to the possible adverse effects. Further prospective randomized studies of ovarian drilling versus ovulation induction are warranted.

REFERENCES

Adelson, M. (1991) Use of the intestinal isolation bag in gynaecological surgery. *Obstet Gynaecol*, **78**, 447–50.

Amar, N.A. and Lachelin, G.C.L. (1993) Laparoscopic ovarian diathermy: an effective treatment for anti-oestrogen resistant anovulatory infertility in women with polycystic ovaries. *Br J Obstet Gynaecol*, **100**, 161–4.

Andolf, E. and Jorgensen, S. (1988) A prospective comparison of clinical ultrasound and operative examination of the female pelvis. *J Ultrasound Med*, **7**, 617–20.

Audebert, A. (1993) Laparoscopic ovarian surgery and ovarian torsion, in *Endoscopic Surgery for Gynaecologists*, (eds. C.J.G. Sutton and M. Diamond), W.B. Saunders, London, pp. 134–41.

Baltarowich, O.H., Kurtz, A.B., Pasto, M.E. *et al.* (1987) The spectrum of sonographic findings in haemorrhagic ovarian cysts. *AJR*, **148**, 901–5.

Bourne, T.H. (1991) Transvaginal color doppler in gynecology. *Ultrasound Obstet Gynecol*, **1**, 359–73.

Bret, P.M., Guibaud, L., Atri, M. *et al.* (1992a) Transvaginal ultrasound-guided aspiration of ovarian cysts and solid pelvic masses. *Radiology*, **185**, 377–80.

Bret, P.M., Atri, M., Guibaud, L. *et al.* (1992b) Ovarian cysts in postmenopausal women; preliminary results with transvaginal alcohol sclerosis. *Radiology*, **184**, 661–3.

Brosens, I. and Puttemans, P. (1989) Double-optic laparoscopy, salpingoscopy, ovrian cystoscopy and endo-ovarian surgery with argon laser, in *Bailliere's Clinical Obstetrics and Gynaecology. Laparoscopic Surgery*, (ed. C.J.G. Sutton), **3**, 595–608.

Bruhat, M.A., Wattiez, A., Mage, G. Pouly, J.L. and Canis, M. (1989) CO$_2$ laser laparoscopy, in *Bailliere's Clinical Obstetrics and Gynaecology. Laparoscopic Surgery*, (ed. C.J.G. Sutton), **3**, 487–97.

Buckman, R.F., Woods, M., Sargent, L. *et al.* (1976) A unifying pathogenic mechanism in the aetiology of intra-peritoneal adhesions. *J Surg Res*, **20**, 1–5.

Buttery, B.W., Beischer, N.A., Fortune, D.W. and Macaffee, C.A.J. (1973) Ovarian tumours in pregnancy. *Med J Austr*, **1**, 345–9.

Canis, M., Mage, G., Wattiez, A. *et al.* (1994) The role of laparoscopic surgery in gynaecology oncology. *Current Opinion Obstet Gynaecol*, **6**, 210–14.

Daniell, J.F., Kurtz, B.R. and Gurley, L.D. (1991) Laser laparoscopic management of large ovarian endometriomas. *Fertil Steril*, **55**, 692–5.

Davis, G.D. and Herubi, P.H. (1989) Transabdominal laser colpotomy. *J Reprod Med*, **34**, 438–40.

De Crespigny, L., Robinson, H.P., Davoren, R.A.M. and Fortune, D.W. (1985) Ultrasound-guided puncture for gynecological and pelvic lesions. *Aust NZ J Obstet Gynaecol*, **25**, 227–9.

Deland, M., Fried, A., Van Nagell, J.R. and Donaldson, E.S. (1979) Ultrasonography in the diagnosis of tumors of the ovary. *Surg Gynecol Obstet*, **148**, 346–8.

Dembo, A.J., Davy, M. and Stenwig, A.E. (1990) Prognostic factor in patients with Stage I epithelial ovarian cancer. *Obstet Gynecol*, **75**, 263–72.

Dewhurst, J. (1981) *Integrated Obstetrics and Gynaecology for Postgraduates*, 3rd edn. Blackwell Scientific, London, pp. 762.

Diernaes, E., Rasmussen, J., Soerensen, T. and Hasch, E. (1987) Ovarian cysts: management by puncture? *Lancet*, **1**, 1084.

Donnez, J., Nisolle, M., Wayembergh, M. *et al.* (1989) CO$_2$ laparoscopy in peritoneal endometriosis and in ovarian endometrial cyst, in *Laser Operative Laparoscopy and Hysteroscopy*, (ed. J. Donnez), Nauwelaerts Printing, Louvain, Belgium, pp. 53–78.

Donnez, J., Nisolle, M., Grandgean, P. *et al.* (1992) The place of GnRH agonists in the treatment of endometriosis and fibroids by advanced endoscopic techniques. *Br J Obstet Gynaecol*, **99**, 31–3.

Dordoni, D., Zaglio, S., Zucca, S. and Favalli, G. (1993) The role of sonographically guided aspiration in the clinical management of ovarian cysts. *J Ultrasound Med*, **12**, 27–31.

Dubuisson, J.B. and Chapron, C. (1994) Complications of dermoid cysts: spillage and dissemination, in *The Management of Adnexal Cysts*, (ed. M.A. Bruhat), Blackwell Scientific, Oxford, pp. 126–30.

Fayez, J.A. and Vogel, M.F. (1991) Comparison of different treatment methods of endometriomas by laparoscopy. *Obstet Gynecol*, **78**, 660–5.

Finkler, N.J., Benacerraf, B., Lavin, P.T. *et al.* (1988) Comparison of serum CA125, clinical impression and ultrasound in the preoperative evaluation of ovarian masses. *Obstet Gynecol*, **72**, 659–64.

Finn, C.B., Luesley, D.M., Buxton, E.J. *et al.* (1992) Is Stage I epithelial ovarian cancer overtreated both surgically and systemically? Results of a five-year cancer registry review. *Br J Obstet Gynaecol*, **99**, 54 8.

Gjonnaess, H. (1984) Polycystic ovarian syndrome

treated by ovarian electro-cautery through the laparoscope. *Fertil Steril*, **41**, 20–5.

Gleeson, N.C., Nicosia, S.V., Mark, J.E., Hoffman, M.S. and Cavanagh, D. (1993) Abdominal wall metastases from ovarian cancer after laparoscopy. *Am J Obstet Gynecol*, **169**, 522–3.

Goldstein, S. and Subramanyam, B. (1989) The postmenopausal cystic adnexal mass: the potential role of ultrasound in conservative management. *Obstet Gynecol*, **73**, 8–12.

Granberg, S., and Wikland, M. (1991) Ultrasound in the diagnosis and treatment of ovarian cystic tumours. *Human Reprod*, **6**, 177–85.

Granberg, S., Wikland, M. and Jansson, I. (1989a) Macroscopic characterisation of ovarian tumours and the relation to the histological diagnosis: criteria to be used for ultrasound evaluation. *Gynecol Oncol*, **35**, 139–44.

Granberg, S., Crona, A., Enk, L. *et al.* (1989b) Ultrasound guided puncture of cystic tumours in the lower pelvis of young women. *J Clin Ultrasound*, **17**, 107–11.

Granberg, S., Norstrom, A. and Wikland, M. (1990) Tumours in the lower pelvis as imaged by vaginal sonography. *Gynecol Oncol*, **37**, 224–9.

Granberg, S., Norstrom, A. and Wikland, M. (1993) Comparison of endovaginal ultrasound and cytological evaluation of cystic ovarian tumours. *J Ultrasound Med*, **12**, 27–31.

Greenblatt, E. (1993) Surgical options in polycystic ovarian syndrome. *Bailliere's Clin Obstet Gynaecol*, **7**, 421–33.

Herrmann, U.J. Jr, Locher, G.W. and Goldhirsch, A. (1987) Sonographic patterns of ovarian tumours: prediction of malignancy. *Obstet Gynecol*, **69**, 777–81.

Hibbard, L.T. (1985) Adnexal torsion. *Am J Obstet Gynecol*, **152**, 456–61.

Hill, L.M., Johnson, C.E. and Lee, R.A. (1975) Ovarian surgery in pregnancy. *Am J Obstet Gynecol*, **122**, 565–9.

Hogston, P. and Lilford, R.J. (1986) Ultrasound study of ovarian cysts in pregnancy: prevalence and significance. *Br J Obstet Gynaecol*, **93**, 625–8.

Johns, D.A. (1993) Laparoscopic treatment of tubo-ovarian abscess, *in Endoscopic Surgery for Gynaecologists*, (eds C.J.G. Sutton and M. Diamond), W.B. Saunders, London, pp. 154–8.

Kane, M.G. and Krejs, G.J. (1984) Complications of diagnostic laparoscopy in Dallas: a 7 year prospective study. *Gastrointest Endosc*, **30**, 237–40.

Kaw, K.T. and Walker, W.J. (1990) Ultrasound guided fine needle aspiration of ovarian cysts: diagnosis and treatment in pregnant and non-pregnant women. *Clin Radiol*, **41**, 105–8.

Kurjak, A. and Predanic, M. (1992) New scoring system for prediction of ovarian malignancy based on transvaginal color doppler sonography. *J Ultrasound Med*, **11**, 631–8.

Livraghi, T., Damascelli, B., Lombard, C. *et al.* (1983) Risk of fine needle abdominal biopsy. *J Clin Ultrasound*, **11**, 77.

Macdonald, R. and Sutton, C.J.G. (1992) Adhesions and laser laparoscopic adhesiolysis, in *Lasers in Gynaecology*, (ed. C.J.G. Sutton), Chapman & Hall, London, pp. 95–118.

Mage, G., Canis, M., Manhes, H. *et al.* (1990) Laparoscopic management of adnexal cystic masses. *J Gynaecol Surg*, **6**, 71–9.

Manhes, H., Canis, M., Wattiez, A. *et al.* (1992) Conservative laparoscopic management of adnexal torsion, in *The Mangement of Adnexal Cysts*, (ed. M.A. Bruhat), Blackwell Scientific, Oxford, pp. 236–41.

Marrs, R.P. (1991) The use of the KTP laser for laparoscopic removal of ovarian endometriomas. *Am J Obstet Gyecol*, **164**, 1622–6.

Meire, H.B. Farrant, P. and Guha, T. (1978) Distinction of benign from malignant ovarian cysts by ultrasound. *Br J Obstet Gynaecol*, **85**, 893–9.

Mintz, M. (1977) Risks and prophylaxis in laparoscopy: a survey of 100000 cases. *J Reprod Med*, **18**, 269–72.

Moyle, J.W., Rochester, D., Sider, L. *et al.* (1983) Sonography of ovarian tumors: predictability of tumour type. *AJR*, **141**, 985–91.

Myerscough, P.R. (1982) *Munro Kerr's Operative Obstetrics*, 10th edn, Baillière Tindall, London, p. 215.

Naether, O.G.J., Fischer, R. and Weise, H.C. (1993) Laparoscopic electrocoagulation of the ovarian surface in infertile patients with polycystic ovarian disease. *Fertil Steril*, **60**, 88–94.

Nezhat, C., Nezhat, F. and Nezhat, C. (1991) Operative laparoscopy (minimally invasive surgery): state of the art. *J Gynaecol Surg*, **8**, 111–41.

Parewijck, W., Thiery, M. and Timperman, J. (1979) Serious complications of laparoscopy. *Med Science Law*, **19**, 199–201.

Peterson, H.B., Hulka, J.F. and Phillips, J.M. (1990) American Association of Gynecologic Laparoscopists' 1988 membership survey on operative laparoscopy. *J Reprod Med*, **35**, 587.

Pinto, M.M., Bernstein, L.H., Brogan, D.A. *et al.* (1990) Measurement of CA-125, carcinoembryonic antigen and alpha-fetoprotein in ovarian cyst fluid: diagnostic adjunct to cytology. *Diagn Cytopathol*, **6**, 160–3.

Reich, H., and McGlynn, F. (1987) Laparoscopic treatment of tubo-ovarian and pelvic abscess. *J Reprod Med*, **32**, 747–50.

Reich, H., McGlynn, F. and Wilkie, W. (1990) Laparoscopic management of Stage I ovarian cancer. A case report. *J Reprod Med*, **35**, 601–5.

Reich, H., De Caprio, J., McGlynn, F. and Taylor, P.J. (1992) Laparoscopic diagnosis and management of acute adnexal torsion. *Gynaecol Endosc*, **2**, 37–8.

Sevelda, P., Vavra, N., Schemper, M. and Salzer, H. (1990) Prognostic factors for survival in Stage I epithelial ovarian carcinoma. *Cancer*, **65**, 2349–52.

Sutton, C.J.G. (1993) Lasers in infertility. *Human Reprod*, **8**, 133–46.

Sutton, C.J.G. (1995) Endometriosis, infertility and reproductive medicine. *Infertil Reprod Med Clin N Am*, **6**, 591–613.

Thurmond, A.S. (1992) Ovarian cysts: will transvaginal alcohol sclerosis help postmenopausal women? *Radiology*, **184**, 605–6.

Toaff, R., Toaff, M.E. and Peyser, M.R. (1976) Infertility following wedge resection of the ovaries. *Am J Obstet Gynecol*, **124**, 92–6.

Way, S. (1946) Ovarian cystectomy of twisted cysts. *Lancet*, **2**, 47–8.

Weiner, Z., Beck, D., Shteiner, M. *et al.* (1993) Screening for ovarian cancer in women with breast cancer with transvaginal sonography and color flow imaging. *J Ultrasound Med*, **12**, 387–93.

Zanetta, G., Trio, D., Lissoni, A. and Dallavalle, C. (1993) Early and short term complications after ultrasound guided puncture of gynecologic lesions: evaluation after 1000 consecutive cases. *Radiology*, **189**, 161–4.

Zweizig, S., Perron, J., Crubb, D. and Mishell, J. (1993) Conservative management of adnexal torsion. *Am J Obstet Gynecol*, **168**, 1791–5.

R.A.F. Crawford and J.H. Shepherd

INTRODUCTION

Operative laparoscopy has progressed dramatically in the last ten years with most operative procedures now having an endoscopic equivalent. Gynecological cancer has attracted the attention of the skilled laparoscopist because of the goal of performing an alternative to open radical surgery without the apparent morbidity. In this chapter, we shall review the endoscopic techniques used for radical surgery in the treatment of early cervix cancer and endometrial cancer. The role of laparoscopic surgery for adnexal masses will be discussed and the complex problems relating to both early and late ovarian cancer and minimal access surgery will be reviewed. The introduction of new techniques must have clear benefit for the patient, in terms of increased cure or decreased morbidity or reduced cost and patient inconvenience. The use of laparoscopic methods solely because they are new and available is not appropriate and we feel that laparoscopy in gynecological cancer management should be modified to complement accepted oncological practice rather than risk a compromise in care.

In minimal access surgery (MAS), it is clear that the cosmetic outcome is better, postoperative analgesic requirement is less, hospitalization can be shorter or even reduced to an outpatient visit, there is a reduced incidence of ileus due to less bowel handling and improved exposure in the true pelvis due to the 10-fold magnification of the laparoscope. The disadvantages of the laparoscopic approach are that it is technically more difficult as an analog of open surgery, the longer operating time needs more theater space, often not available in the busy National Health Service in the UK or in Canada. Controversies in surgical oncology and laparoscopy include the radicality of resection compared to the standard operation and contamination of ports and other sites related to specimen handling and retrieval.

The operation which has been successfully adapted for the laparoscopic route is the lymphadenectomy. Both pelvic and para-aortic lymphadenectomy are possible. The indications for this surgery have changed in the last decade with the advent of surgical staging of ovarian and endometrial cancer and the resurgence of surgery for early carcinoma of the cervix. The laparoscopist should only consider this operation if properly trained in oncological surgery. There can be significant morbidity attached to a lymphadenectomy, both in the short term with hemorrhage and nerve damage and in the long term with lymphocyst and lymphedema formation.

OPEN LYMPHADENECTOMY

Meigs added the pelvic lymphadenectomy to the Wertheim's radical hysterectomy as one of his modifications and the pelvic lympha-

Gynecological Endoscopic Surgery. Edited by C.J.G. Sutton. Published in 1997 by Chapman & Hall, London. ISBN 0 412 58040 3.

denectomy is still performed as part of the surgical treatment of early carcinoma of the cervix. The percentage of positive lymph node metastases to the pelvic lymph nodes in stage Ib disease ranges from 9% (Artman *et al.*, 1987) to 31% (Burghardt *et al.*, 1987). An overview of reports containing more than 1000 patients gave an average of 17% with positive lymph nodes (Hoskins, 1988). A low para-aortic (below the inferior mesenteric artery) lymphadenectomy may be considered to be part of the procedure as 7.5% of stage Ib carcinomas have metastatic disease in the para-aortic nodes (Winter *et al.*, 1988) especially in stage Ibii tumors (Patsner *et al.*, 1992). Women who have positive pelvic nodes after radical surgery for cervix cancer will be offered radiotherapy for control of pelvic recurrence (Remy *et al.*, 1990). Although they have had the central tumor debulked and a complete pelvic lymphadenectomy, these women will suffer increased morbidity relating to their combination treatment. The urinary fistula and bowel obstruction rate in those women with a large tumor removed by radical surgery followed by treatment with adjuvant radiotherapy is 14.2% (Bloss *et al.*, 1992). Postoperative radiotherapy for women with node-positive disease does not improve survival (Morrow, 1980). In endometrial and ovarian cancer, the lymphatic spread is both to the high (above the inferior mesenteric artery up to the renal vessels) and low para-aortic areas (below the inferior mesenteric artery).

The technique employed for an open para-aortic lymphadenectomy is similar to that described by Oram and Bridges (1987). The abdomen is opened in an extended midline incision. After a thorough laparotomy, the small bowel is packed away in the upper abdomen. A broad-bladed retractor is placed with its tip under the third part of the duodenum to aid exposure. The para-aortic region is palpated and two stay sutures are placed in the retroperitoneum overlying the aorta about 5 cm above the bifurcation. A midline incision is made between the stay sutures and the loose areolar tissue is divided. The landmarks are clearly identified (the aorta, the inferior vena cava and the ureters). The fatty nodal tissue is picked up with tissue forceps and, using a mixture of sharp and blunt dissection with diathermy and titanium clips (Liga) for the hemostasis, samples of nodal tissue are removed. Care is taken to avoid damaging the sympathetic chain. Tissue is taken as far up as the third part of the duodenum which is the limit of the dissection. Some authors (Winter *et al.*, 1988) who favor a lymphadenectomy of this area up to the renal vessels suggest ligating and dividing the inferior mesenteric artery to avoid accidental damage to this vessel. Following hemostasis, the peritoneum is closed using a dissolvable suture. The retroperitoneal dissection often leads to a significant ileus and therefore the stomach is drained for 24–48 hours using a nasogastric tube. The position of this tube is checked at laparotomy.

The pelvic lymphadenectomy is then performed as follows. The pelvic side wall is approached by dividing the round ligament and separating the areolar tissue overlying the great vessels. The paravesical space is formed anteriorly and the pararectal space posteriorly. At this time, the ureter is clearly seen on the medial leaf of the peritoneum. If an oophorectomy is to be carried out, then the infundibulopelvic ligament would be ligated and divided. Care must be taken that the ureter is not included in this bundle. The ureter is dissected from the peritoneum and supported with a soft rubber sling. The pelvic lymphadenectomy is started by sweeping the fatty lymphatic tissue from the adventitia of the external iliac vessels, having divided the chain at its distal margin, the superficial circumflex iliac vein. A mixture of hemostatic clips and diathermy is used for both hemostasis and lymphostasis. The space behind the external iliac artery and between the artery and vein are exposed to insure that no nodal tissue is missed. During the dissection of the external iliac group of lymph nodes, the genitofemoral nerve is clearly identified. It would only be sacrificed if it was involved in obviously malignant nodes. The retroperitoneal space is opened further cranially and the lymphatic tissue overlying the common iliac artery is then also removed. Care is taken not to damage the ureter at this level.

The external iliac vein is carefully retracted using a vein retractor and the obturator fossa is viewed. Using a mixture of palpation and direct vision, the obturator nerve is identified and the bundle of lymphatic tissue is separated from the nerve. Using a Babcock forceps, this cord of tissue is then peeled off the side wall of the pelvis, away from the obturator nerve and removed after hemostatic clips have been applied. This tissue comprises both the deep and superficial obturator group of nodes and is perhaps the most important lymph node group to be sampled in cervical cancer. Occasionally, an aberrant obturator vessel can give rise to substantial hemorrhage. Around the internal iliac artery, the lymph nodes removed comprise the internal iliac group. Occasionally, this sample is small and the remaining nodes of this group will be included in any lymphatic tissue with the uterine artery. Hemostasis is obtained using diathermy and Liga clips. The use of a hot pack can reduce venous ooze. Damage to the great vessels is repaired immediately using fine (5-0) Prolene sutures. The process of the pelvic lymphadenectomy can be aided by tilting the table approximately 15° away from the operator. FIGO stated a radical lymphadenectomy must yield at least 20 nodes (Ferraris *et al.*, 1988). However, apart from the quality of surgery, the node count is also dependent on factors such as the woman's anatomy and the technique of pathological assessment.

The use of frozen section in assessing lymph node was reviewed by Bjornsson *et al.* (1993). The sensitivity of frozen section as compared to paraffin section was 68% with a specificity of 100%. The only metastases missed by frozen section were less than 2 mm in size, although all these nodes were regarded as suspicious on palpation by a pathologist. The use of lymphangiography to indicate pelvic lymph node involvement is not entirely reliable (Stellato *et al.*, 1992). In women with small cervical tumors (<3 cm) with impalpable para-aortic nodes, the preaortic retroperitoneal space is not opened because of the unnecessary morbidity. This practice is supported by the evidence from Patsner *et al.* (1992), where in 125 cases of small tumors (less than 3 cm) there were only two positive para-aortic nodes. Both these cases had grossly positive pelvic nodes.

The use of peritoneal cytology is well known in the staging of ovarian cancer and has recently been introduced into the staging of endometrial cancer. In the surgical management of early cervical cancer, peritoneal washings are of no value (Morris *et al.*, 1992).

Following pelvic lymphadenectomy, it is our practice to use a closed suction drain which is left *in situ* for 7–10 days or until there have been two consecutive days with less than 20 ml drainage. Prospective trials have shown that drainage of the pelvic side walls does not decrease lymphocyst formation (Barton *et al.*, 1992) although the use of drains was also introduced to reduce fistula formation.

It is a matter of personal preference as to whether the pelvic lymphadenectomy at open operation is performed before or after the radical hysterectomy.

LAPAROSCOPIC PELVIC LYMPHADENECTOMY

With the advent of advanced laparoscopic equipment that allows accurate manipulation and dissection of tissue and good hemostasis, the laparoscopic lymphadenectomy is becoming an acceptable operation. The laparoscopic lymphadenectomy procedure can allow the full staging of the abdomen and aid a radical vaginal approach for the treatment of the primary tumor. It is entirely feasible to use the techniques to perform an adequate staging of early ovarian cancer (pelvic an para-aortic lymph node sampling, peritoneal washings and multiple biopsies from around the abdomen; Querleu and Leblanc (1994); Childers *et al.* (1995)) although the management of the primary tumor may be less than adequate.

Transperitoneal laparoscopic pelvic lymphadenectomy was described in 1991 (Querleu *et al.*, 1991). The two monitors are placed just beyond the patient's feet, allowing a comfortable operating position for the two surgeons. The bladder is kept empty with a Foley catheter. The technique involves using a camera mounted on a 10 mm 0° laparoscope which is placed through a subumbilical incision. Three further ports are used for manipulation, dissection, hemostasis via diathermy or ligation and specimen retrieval. Two 5 mm ports are used in the iliac fossae and a 10–12 mm port is used in the midline suprapubic area. This larger port allows the use of a Ligaclip applicator or linear stapler/cutter device and also allows retrieval of the tissue. Placement of these instrument ports should not be too low as this can restrict their use on the side wall. The 5 mm ports are placed laterally to allow a good angle for operating on the contralateral side.

As usual for operative laparoscopy, a thorough inspection of the abdomen is performed. In cases of endometrial and ovarian cancer, washings for cytology are taken. A steep Trendelenburg position allows the small bowel to be moved out of the pelvis. A nasogastric tube insures that the stomach is emptied of any gas, allowing more space in the upper abdomen for the bowel. The round ligament is elevated and divided with diathermy to access the pelvic side wall. If the lymphadenectomy is diagnostic with the uterus being left *in situ*, this division of the round ligament is not essential. We use monopolar disposable scissors for this maneuver. The use of a disposable instrument insures reliable insulation of the shaft and dependable sharpness of the blades. Using the scissors and a blunt dissector, the external iliac

artery and vein on the side wall are visualized. The temptation is to begin the dissection too far laterally and this will lead to damage to the genitofemoral nerve and psoas muscle. Once the major vessels are exposed and the surgeon is correctly orientated, the sheath of fat containing the nodal tissue can be stripped cleanly. Diathermy is used to maintain hemostasis. It is important to avoid bleeding as the staining of the tissues obscures the view as well as reducing the light available. Due to the magnifying effect of the laparoscope, good views are obtained, allowing accurate hemostasis to be achieved. The paravesical and pararectal spaces are developed with blunt dissection as in the open lymphadenectomy.

The obturator fossa is easily identified by slipping medially over the external iliac vein. The obturator nerve is identified at the caudal end and the nodal bundle is teased out of the fossa using a mixture of traction and sharp dissection with diathermy. Attention is paid to preserving the obturator nerve by identifying it before any sharp dissection or cautery is performed. If the nodal dissection is approached from the cranial end there is considerable danger of dividing the nerve as it leaves the muscle. Diathermy and occasionally Ligaclips are used especially if an aberrant obturator vessel is damaged. Tamponade is useful to enable a clear view if a large vessel is damaged and this may be achieved using a tonsillar swab (gauze approximately 1 cm × 6 cm). These swabs can be easily retrieved with a laparoscopic Babcock's forceps. The repair of injuries caused to vessels and structures during laparoscopy can be performed either using laparoscopic techniques or via a standard open method and this is left to the discretion and experience of the operator.

At present we remove our lymphatic samples through the 10–12 mm port using the laparoscopic Babcock's forceps. We favor a clear plastic port with a flap valve which allows a good view of the sample as it is removed from biopsy site to the outside. Alternatively, a Ceolio-extractor, a three-pronged retracting forceps (Lépine, Lyon, France), can be used to retrieve the tissue. The contamination of portal site with malignant tissue is a potential problem but in squamous cancer of the cervix, this has not figured in the literature except in one case (Fidalgo de Matos *et al.*, 1993). The pelvic lymphadenectomy, including the division of the ovarian and uterine pedicles, takes two hours.

LAPAROSCOPIC PARA-AORTIC LYMPHADENECTOMY

Para-aortic lymphadenectomy has a role in endometrial, ovarian and some cases of cervical cancer. Para-aortic lymph node sampling was first described in 1993 by Querleu. The main difficulty encountered with this surgery using the laparoscope is that the small bowel can obscure the field. As with the pelvic lympadenectomy, the surgeon should be clear about the indications for the surgery as well as competent to perform the open surgery before embarking on this process laparoscopically.

The mesentery of the small bowel should be identified and bowel splayed across the abdomen to the left upper quadrant. A steep Trendelenburg position is required for this surgery and it is prudent to warn the anesthetist so that they can insure adequate protection of the patient and prevent slippage on the operating table. The two monitor screens are placed at the level of the patient's shoulders on either side so that the surgeon and assistant can work comfortably. Identification of the landmarks is essential prior to laparoscopic surgery in the retroperitoneum. The transverse or third part of the duodenum is visualized crossing the inferior vena cava and aorta and caudally the ureter is identified crossing the bifurcation of the iliac vessels. The right-sided para-aortic lymphadenectomy is performed with the surgeon standing on the left of the patient with scissors through the left lateral port and graspers through the lower midline port. The assistant, standing on the patient's right, holds the camera and telescope

through the subumbilical port and another pair of graspers through the right lateral port. Therefore, the same ports are used for both the pelvic and para-aortic parts of the surgery. It is sometimes helpful to rotate the camera through 90° so that the great vessels appear horizontal on the screen.

An incision is made over the aorta between the mesentery of the small bowel and the right common iliac artery. This allows access from the upper external iliac artery to the transverse duodenum. The peritoneum is lifted and blunt dissection is performed laterally until the ureter is identified. This is then dissected free from the underlying tissue and reflected laterally. By placing the graspers underneath the ureter and retracting laterally the peritoneum forms a cover protecting the operating field from coils of small bowel. As in the open lympadenectomy, the nodal tissue is removed by finding the adventitia of the aorta with sharp dissection and carefully removing the fat containing the lymph nodes, using bipolar diathermy for hemostasis. Attention needs to be paid to the perforating vessels from both the aorta and vena cava. Ligaclips are probably advised for the larger vessels and these can be applied using the disposable multifire applicator which will fit through the midline port. It is useful to clip the top end of the dissection for later radiological identification as well as hemo- and lymphostasis. Careful inspection of the area aided by judicious cautery confirms hemostasis.

The nodal package is then brought out through the midline port as previously described. The left-sided dissection is performed with the surgeon standing on the patient's right utilizing the instruments (scissors and graspers) through the midline and right lateral ports. The left-sided dissection is performed in a similar manner to that previously described except that the plane along the aorta is developed before the lateral dissection. Attention is drawn to the origin of the inferior mesenteric artery as it can be easily damaged and lead to major hemorrhage. The adventitia over the aorta is cleared and then the psoas muscle is exposed laterally. This procedure allows the surgeon to displace the ureter forward and thus protect it. The assistant places the grasper under this ureter and rectosigmoid mesentery allowing the surgeon to dissect out the left sided para-aortic bundle in safety. The nodal bundle is elevated and separated with a mixture of sharp and blunt dissection. The cephalad end is divided and the nodal strip is brought down. It can either be divided at the caudal end or the dissection can continue into the left common iliac group of nodes. The sample is then removed through the midline portal.

Fowler *et al.* (1993) compared the yield from the laparoscopic approach with an open lymphadenectomy. In this study, between 62% and 97% of the total lymph nodes removed were sampled laparoscopically. Total lymph nodes removed at open operation ranged from 11 to 46, with between seven and 33 being removed laparoscopically. However, the authors point out that there is a significant learning curve with this procedure and the percentage recovered laparoscopically in the second half of their series was significantly greater than in the first half (85% versus 63%, p < 0.005). Interestingly, no patient with negative nodes at laparoscopy had positive pelvic nodes found at laparotomy. Another group (Childers *et al.*, 1992) reported a 91% yield in lymph nodes removed laparoscopically, compared with that at laparotomy. Spirtos *et al.* (1995) reported an average of 20.8 pelvic and 7.9 para-aortic lymph nodes per patient in their paper. An Australian study (Johnson *et al.*, 1994) demonstrated that in the porcine model, the laparoscopic lymphadenectomy was equivalent to the open operation. In patients, however, the same surgeon did not find the operations were similar, with the laparoscopic approach being inferior (Johnson, 1994).

The role of a therapeutic lymphadenectomy performed laparoscopically in the management of cervical cancer is still controversial although it appears that an adequate diagnostic procedure is entirely feasible. Our view is that a lymphadenectomy will demonstrate the absence of lymph node metastases and therefore allow a less morbid but equally radical vaginal procedure in the management of early cervix cancer. Downey *et al.* (1989) suggested that the surgical clearance of macroscopically involved pelvic nodes in the 41% of their patients with stage Ib–IIa cervical cancer with positive nodes had a survival benefit. This point is disputed by Potter *et al.* (1990) as there was no survival benefit in their study when completion of the radical hysterectomy in the presence of metastatic lymph nodes with adjuvant radiotherapy was compared to abandoning the surgery, leaving the uterus *in situ* for easier application of the postoperative radiotherapy.

As there are few reports published to date on laparoscopic lymphadenectomy, it is not known what effect the laparoscopic management has on the morbidity of subsequent treatment. There is a learning curve for the laparoscopic procedure and the operating time can be protracted. The length of procedure and the presence of insufflated gas may also have an effect on implantation of tumor at distant sites. The transperitoneal laparoscopic approach for lymphadenectomy in cervical cancer (described above) appears to have less morbidity (1.9% of 301 cases) compared to the laparoscopic retroperitoneal approach (28% of 200 cases) (Fidalgo de Matos *et al.*, 1993) and fewer adhesions than the open retroperitoneal route (Fowler *et al.*, 1994). Interestingly, the reported morbidity from the USA using the same transperitoneal operation in relation to prostate cancer is higher (15% of 362 cases) (Kavoussi *et al.*, 1993).

CERVICAL CANCER

The role of laparoscopic surgery in the management of early cervical cancer has an exciting potential. However, it must be viewed with caution as we remember that conventional surgery has a relatively low morbidity rate and a high cure rate. The trade-off for the reduced hospital stay and cosmetic scar must not be at the cost of cancer recurrence or higher morbidity. Some leaders in this field suggest that the lymphadenectomy can become part of the staging procedure allowing the doctor to proceed with radical surgery if the women are node negative. At present, we do not send our lymphadenectomy specimen for frozen section and perform the operation at the same time as the radical vaginal surgery.

We favor the use of radical vaginal surgery in conjunction with laparoscopy as pioneered in France rather than the total laparoscopic approach favored by some in the USA. The pelvic and para-aortic (if required) lymphadenectomy is performed laparoscopically as described. A bilateral oophorectomy is performed as per the usual indications (a poorly differentiated tumor, adenocarcinoma or age over 40 years). The infundibulopelvic ligament is ligated or clipped after the ureter has been clearly demonstrated. The pedicle is then cut with diathermy scissors and a loop tie is placed over the pedicle. Alternatively, a linear stapler can be used for the infundibulopelvic ligament. The uterine artery is divided at its origin. Either clips or staples can be used in this situation. Dargent favors the use of the linear stapler cutter to divide the uterine artery and upper portion of the cardinal ligaments (Dargent *et al.*, 1994). He then places a further staple line down to the pelvic floor laterally on these ligaments. The bottom end of this staple line is then grasped from below when the Schauta hysterectomy is completed. The division of the uterine artery early and laterally allows an easier, almost blood-free radical vaginal hysterectomy.

The Schauta hysterectomy is seldom taught in the UK and there are few with a wide experience in this technique. The vaginal cuff is formed and then closed over the tumor. We have found that with adequate retraction and laparoscopic preparation, a Schuhardt incision is seldom required. Vaginal side wall retrac-

tors of various widths and lengths are available which greatly facilitate this operation. The bladder is reflected in the midline and the bladder pillars are developed. The ureter is then dissected free from these pillars using careful palpation and sharp dissection. This maneuver is similar to the deroofing of the ureteric tunnel during the classic Wertheim hysterectomy. The ureter is then retracted out of the way and the uterine artery lies in view. As this has been divided laterally, it is bloodless. The uterosacral ligaments are then divided flush on the rectum as in Wertheim's hysterectomy. By using traction on the first clamp on the cardinal ligaments, the second clamp can be applied more laterally, insuring a good 2 cm of paracolpos with the specimen. The bottom of the staple line is then found and completes the removal of the paracolpos. It is this paracervical tissue which is the key to the operation and it is this very area where the laparoscopic radical hysterectomy is deficient. We do not place any drains and the bladder is catheterized for up to two weeks. The radical dissection around the bladder base and ureters and uterosacral ligaments leads to a degree of bladder dysfunction which resolves rapidly. It is, however, prudent to drain the bladder to reduce infection and other urinary problems such as fistulae.

The laparoscopic radical hysterectomy follows the steps of the open radical hysterectomy. The ureter is dissected free and its tunnel deroofed. The bladder is reflected and the uterosacral and lateral ligaments divided using staple guns. However, the paracolpos remains difficult to approach via the laparoscope. The complication rate of this approach is unacceptably high even taking into account the learning of a new operation (4/6 had significant bladder or ureteric injuries; Sedlacek *et al.* (1995)).

In certain cases of squamous cell cancer, it may be possible to conserve the uterus for future childbearing. We have had limited experience of this (five cases) but Professor Dargent has reported a series of 28 cases (Dargent *et al.*,

1994). In this series, there have been ten pregnancies with five live births and one recurrence which occurred in the para-aortic region. Essentially, if there is a small exophytic cancer and it is possible to obtain a good cancer-free margin below the internal os, the uterus can remain *in situ*. The pelvic lymph nodes are assessed laparoscopically. A cervical suture of a non-absorbable monofilament (1-0 nylon) is inserted at the isthmus and buried under the vaginoisthmic epithelium. This is to prevent cervical incompetence in subsequent pregnancies and its accurate placement at the original operation is important.

The use of operative laparoscopy in the management of recurrent cervical cancer offers a potential method for improving selection of cases which would benefit from exenterative surgery. CT scanning can be used to determine those cases where further radical surgery can be curative (Crawford *et al.*, 1996). In a case report of three patients, Plante and Roy (1995) describe the use of laparoscopy to identify inoperable recurrence, saving the women unnecessary surgery.

ENDOMETRIAL CANCER

Endometrial cancer is the commonest gynecological cancer in the USA and the second most common pelvic malignancy in the UK and its incidence is increasing (Oram, 1990). The five-year overall survival rate is only 67% (Kottmaier, 1982) even though 75% of women present with stage I disease. The classic presenting symptom of endometrial cancer is postmenopausal bleeding. The underlying reason for the overall low survival rate is that the state of health of these women is generally poor and only 50% of cases are suitable for extensive surgery (Lees, 1978; Nahhas *et al.*, 1980). In 1988, FIGO issued new staging guidelines for endometrial cancer (Shepherd, 1989) based on a surgical appraisal of the cancer and its spread rather than a clinical assessment under anesthetic. This change was because of the discrepancy in clinical stage if

there was pre-existing uterine enlargement and reflected that the majority of endometrial cancers are treated surgically due to their early presentation.

Endometrial cancer is usually treated with a simple total abdominal hysterectomy and bilateral salpingo-oophorectomy (TAH and BSO) by the general gynecologist. However, stage for stage, the outcome is similar to that of carcinoma of the cervix. The Gynecological Oncology Group (Creaseman *et al.*, 1987) reported 22% extrauterine spread of disease in clinical stage I disease. The FIGO surgical staging requires information to be collected which is not usually available from the records of a simple TAH and BSO. The use of peritoneal washings and assessment of the pelvic and para-aortic lymph nodes should be standard for the complete operation. Homesley *et al.* (1992) reported that this added complexity of surgery does not automatically increase the morbidity of the operation. However, this study was performed by appropriately trained gynecological oncologists. The results of this more extensive and complete surgical staging can alter the type and extent of adjuvant radiotherapy. The basis for this apparently aggressive staging in endometrial cancer is to provide an accurate prognosis (Creaseman *et al.*, 1987). Lymph node involvement in clinical stage I patients ranges from 2% in well-differentiated lesions to 34% in poorly differentiated cancers.

The necessary surgical management in endometrial cancer is accurate staging, resection of the primary tumor and removal of the ovaries. In the staging, peritoneal washings are required for cytology and an assessment of the lymph nodes in the pelvic and para-aortic region necessitates a lymphadenectomy. The central tumor needs to be removed by a simple or extended hysterectomy. It is advisable to remove the ovaries at the same operation as these tumors are hormone dependent. The use of laparoscopy in the surgical management of endometrial cancer allows the staging process to be completed. Peritoneal cytology is easily obtained and the pelvic and para-aortic lymphadenectomy are performed as already described. The removal of the uterus vaginally appears to be ideal. However, there are several factors which have militated against the use of this route routinely prior to operative laparoscopy. There was no way to assess the intra-abdominal organs or lymph nodes for pathology via the vagina alone. This is easily overcome using a laparoscopic procedure. It was not always easy to remove the ovaries via the vagina. Again, laparoscopic preparation allows their consistent and complete removal safely. Finally, a number of these women have narrowed vaginas, making the surgery unnecessarily difficult. The laparoscopic preparation and division of the pedicles from above allows the uterus to be delivered vaginally.

The place of simple vaginal hysterectomy without laparoscopic support was discussed by Peters *et al.* (1983) where a series of cases was presented demonstrating the effectiveness of removing the primary tumor alone. Overall, the five-year survival rate was 94% even though these women were poor operative risks due to their obesity, hypertension or diabetes. A further series (Massi *et al.*, 1996) suggests that vaginal hysterectomy (with bilateral salpingo-oophorectomy in 177/180 cases) is suitable treatment for stage I disease compared to abdominal hysterectomy.

Laparoscopically assisted simple hysterectomy has been well described for benign disease (Reich *et al.*, 1989; Mage *et al.*, 1990; Liu, 1992). The combination of treatment of the primary disease by hysterectomy, the removal of a possible source of hormonal drive by bilateral oophorectomy and accurate staging including peritoneal washings and pelvic and para-aortic lymphadenectomy is sound by modern oncological standards. Childers *et al.* (1993a) presented a schema for the management of endometrial cancer involving laparoscopy. Laparoscopic evaluation was performed on cases which were clinically stage I. If there was no intraperitoneal disease, then a simple laparoscopic-assisted vaginal hyster-

ectomy (LAVH) with bilateral salpingo-oophorectomy was performed. The procedure was then terminated if there was only minimal invasion and the tumor was well differentiated (stage Ia, G1). If the grade of tumor was less than well differentiated, a lymphadenectomy was performed. In the well-differentiated tumor, the LAVH was performed first and a lymphadenectomy was carried out if there was deep myometrial invasion as seen on frozen section. The advantage of the combined laparoscopic approach is the reduced morbidity of the vaginal hysterectomy with the additional removal of the adnexae and a complete staging procedure. The operation can be tailored to the individual woman by not performing the lymphadenectomy in cases with well-differentiated superficial tumors where the likelihood of metastases is low. In Childers' series, there were metastases in the omentum, right hemidiaphragm and para-aortic nodes in patients thought clinically to have stage I disease. This reinforces the point that these women need to have a thorough evaluation of the peritoneal cavity. The management dilemma is, therefore, whether these women should have their disease assessed and treated by laparoscopy or via an extended midline incision. There is no place for the small cosmetic suprapubic transverse incision.

The question remains whether the woman with endometrial cancer should have the added morbidity of the full surgical staging as described by FIGO with pelvic and para-aortic lymphadenectomy. The addition of an open lymphadenectomy appears not to increase the morbidity when performed by an appropriately trained surgeon (Homesley *et al.*, 1992). The need to perform a para-aortic lymphadenectomy has been questioned by Faught *et al.* (1994). This report reviewed 273 patients who had a pelvic lymphadenectomy but no para-aortic lymphadenectomy as part of their staging for endometrial cancer. As there were only 1.5% with distant spread, the authors concluded that there was insufficient evidence to support routine para-aortic node sampling.

This makes the laparoscopic assessment much easier as there is less technical difficulty in only sampling the pelvic nodes prior to the vaginal hysterectomy. At present, we would offer a woman with stage I (clinical) endometrial cancer a LAVH and staging with peritoneal cytology and lymphadenectomy. In recently published management guidelines, Homesley (1996) states that laparoscopic surgery for endometrial carcinoma is an acceptable alternative. A Gynecological Oncology Group trial is examining the value of this procedure compared to the open technique. In an attempt to standardize the operative procedure, the steering committee vets the laparoscopic competence of contributors via videotape as well as reviewing the video of each procedure entered in the trial.

ADNEXAL MASS SURGERY

Laparoscopic adnexal surgery has developed considerably and spread widely since it was first described (Reich, 1987; Nezhat *et al.*, 1989). Aware of the possible dangers of removing early ovarian cancers laparoscopically and therefore possibly compromising patient survival, gynecologists have relied heavily on preoperative ultrasound scanning and serum tumor marker estimation to select benign cases for this procedure. Most gynecologists would perform a laparotomy via a midline incision if there is a suspicion of malignancy. The incidence of malignant cysts occurring in patients where preoperative investigations wrongly suggested that the mass was benign ranges from 0.04% to 3.7% (Peterson *et al.*, 1990; Dressler, 1991; Lehmann-Willenbrock *et al.*, 1991; Hulka *et al.*, 1992; Nezhat *et al.*, 1992; Canis *et al.*, 1994). More recently, there are reports (Reich *et al.*, 1990; Querleu and LeBlanc, 1994; Childers *et al.*, 1995) of surgical staging being performed laparoscopically which includes peritoneal cytology, multiple biopsies, para-aortic and pelvic lymphadenectomy. These reports include both patients with early disease diagnosed at other hospitals and referred for staging and management and a group of women undergoing second-look surgery.

The level of expertise required for laparoscopic adnexectomy or oophorectomy is similar to that for laparoscopic treatment of ectopic pregnancy (RCOG, 1994). In the USA, management of ovarian cysts is the third most common indication for operative laparoscopy (Peterson *et al.*, 1990). Appropriate patient selection is important to avoid operating on malignant masses unwittingly. A survey that we recently carried out (Crawford *et al.*, 1995) indicates that the majority of consultants feel that ultrasound scan (USS) should always be used prior to operation and only 14% operate on clinically palpable lesions alone without the aid of preoperative USS. Color flow Doppler scanning was available to most gynecologists who have an interest in ovarian cancer. In response to the question whether an abnormally increased blood flow in an adnexal mass would reduce use of minimal access surgery (MAS), 23% replied that it would not affect their management. This group of gynecologists had both access to and experience with MAS, suggesting that some gynecologists use MAS even though they suspect a cyst is malignant. Indeed, one gynecologist replied that he would aspirate a cyst showing increased vascularity and send the fluid for cytology, even though cyst cytology is known for false-negative results (Nicklin *et al.*, 1994). CA125 and other tumor markers may be helpful in screening adnexal masses. Only 54% of consultants performed a screening serum CA125 estimation on all adnexal masses. It was used selectively by 42% when they suspected patients had a malignant mass and, therefore, they were not using it as a screening test. A risk score, based on CA125 and USS, has shown high sensitivity (Davies *et al.*, 1993) for predicting ovarian cancer in a woman with an adnexal mass and it would be prudent to know the CA125 result and the USS report prior to MAS. A family history of ovarian cancer can lead to an increased worry for the patient with an adnexal mass and pressure on the clinician to remove it. This is due to an increased lifetime risk of ovarian cancer in these patients. The risk is up to 5% in women with a first-degree relative with ovarian cancer (Kerlikowske *et al.*, 1992). The majority of the consultants surveyed felt that a positive family history is a contraindication to MAS for adnexal masses.

The use of frozen section during MAS has been advocated (Parker and Berek, 1993). In most settings, the use of frozen section for a representative sampling of a cyst would not give a definitive result in time to alter the management on the operating table and it can be misleading, especially in borderline malignancy.

Ultrasound appearances such as the absence of irregular solid parts, thick septa, ascites or matted bowel with a cyst diameter less than 8–10 cm suggest a benign lesion (Herrman *et al.*, 1987; Parker, 1992). American College of Obstetricians and Gynecologists guidelines for MAS detail that the adnexal mass should be less than 10 cm diameter, cystic with a distinct border with no solid parts and there should be no associated ascites or matted bowel, a normal CA125 (<35 U/ml) and no family history of ovarian cancer. As a result of our survey, we suggest the following guidelines for laparoscopic management of adnexal masses:

1. a preoperative USS should be performed; if the USS reveals solid elements, multiloculated areas, a diameter greater than 8 cm, bilateral cysts or increased vascularity on Doppler then MAS should not be performed;
2. a preoperative CA125 should be taken and if raised, caution should be exercised before proceeding with MAS;
3. a family history is a contraindication to MAS for adnexal masses;
4. adnexal masses should be removed completely and, if possible, without rupture whether with MAS or at open operation.

If all adnexal masses are managed laparoscopically irrespective of ultrasound appearances and CA125 levels, the incidence of carcinoma increases to 14% (Childers *et al.* 1996). We feel that based on our current knowledge MAS without reference to USS and tumor markers is unwise. Feasibility of a procedure alone does not justify its use. It is important that there is a consensus view regarding the role of this procedure in the management of adnexal masses and who should be performing it.

The laparoscopic management of endometriotic cysts has been well described. Interestingly, there is now molecular biological evidence (X-inactivation) to show that at least some endometriomas are neoplastic (Nilbert *et al.*, 1995). Taken in conjunction with an estimation that 20% of endometrioid ovarian adenocarcinomas arise from focal malignant changes in ovarian endometriosis (Fox, 1993), this would suggest that both caution and great care be exercised when removing endometriomas.

OVARIAN CANCER

A review of 29 patients (Crawford *et al.*, 1995) who underwent MAS at their referring hospital as part of their initial management was carried out. In 1993, this type of case represented 4.1% (10/243) of our referrals at the Royal Marsden Hospital, Chelsea. The median age of the patients was 37 years (range 20–68). Twenty-five women were premenopausal and 14 were nulliparous. In 17 cases, MAS was performed electively and in the remaining cases MAS was performed as an emergency. It appears that malignancy was suspected at the original MAS in 12 cases. In this group, none of the patients had an immediate laparotomy for staging. The FIGO stage distribution was stage I in 13 patients, stage II in four patients and stage III in 12 patients.

In our survey, the use of MAS in the initial management of ovarian cancer was not confined to any particular stage and patients with early-stage curable ovarian cancer and advanced disease were seen. The accepted current surgical practice for staging ovarian cancer combines a laparotomy via a long midline incision with peritoneal cytology, multiple biopsies and a pelvic and para-aortic lymphadenectomy (Shepherd, 1990). The use of an appropriate incision suggests that the consultants surveyed are performing an adequate staging procedure. Although it is possible to perform the retroperitoneal dissection laparoscopically (Querleu and LeBlanc, 1994) and carry out all the maneuvers required for the FIGO surgical staging of ovarian cancer, it is not known if MAS is as effective as accepted standard practice. Twelve patients in our survey had advanced disease but it was not clear whether this was suspected prior to laparoscopy. The age range of the cases reviewed suggests that gynecologists concerned did not view increasing years as a contraindication to MAS. The use of an age limit such as the menopause to restrict the use of MAS in order to avoid operating on women with malignancy has been challenged (Levine, 1990; Parker and Berek, 1990). They demonstrated that with careful selection, benign lesions could be removed from postmenopausal women with minimal morbidity although both papers had only small numbers of cases. From our cases, it would appear that there is no clear age limit under which clinicians could operate safely without fear of removing a malignant mass unexpectedly.

Surgery for early-stage ovarian cancer is potentially curative and so laparoscopy, if it includes accidental spillage, cyst rupture and incomplete removal, may be detrimental. It is not clear that intraoperative cyst rupture leads to a poorer prognosis. Sevelda *et al.* (1989), Dembo *et al.* (1990), Finn *et al.* (1992), Vergote *et al.* (1993), Sjövall *et al.* (1994) and data from our unit suggest that factors other than cyst rupture at operation are poor prognostic indicators. However, others (Webb *et al.*, 1973; Sainz de la Cuesta *et al.*, 1994) maintain that the intraoperative rupture may specifically worsen prognosis. In the event of intraoperative rupture of a malignant cyst, whether at laparoscopy or at an open procedure, the pelvis and abdomen should be copiously lavaged and the staging with definitive treatment performed as soon as practically possible (Seltzer, 1993), preferably under the same anesthetic. Likewise, if frozen section is used in MAS and malignancy is confirmed, the definitive staging and surgery should be performed immediately. Those gynecologists with most experience in laparoscopic oncology advocate early treatment with adjuvant chemotherapy.

In our series, the delay between the initial MAS and the surgical staging operation was 6.5 weeks which compared to a delay of 4.8 weeks in the Society of Gynecologic Oncologists survey in 1990 (Maiman *et al.*, 1991). A survey performed in Germany suggested that this delay between laparoscopy and staging and definitive treatment may be important in relation to progression of disease (Kindermann *et al.*, 1995). Concern has been raised regarding implantation of tumor in portal sites in ovarian cancer (Shepherd *et al.*, 1994) and other cancers (Cirocco *et al.*, 1994). This may be due to the traumatic delivery of malignant tissue through the minimal access portal or related to other factors such as the increased intra-abdominal pressure. If this implantation occurs and the definitive staging procedure and treatment is delayed, the prognosis may be drastically altered from good (early stage) to poor (stage III or even stage IV, requiring chemotherapy). It is probably this delay in treatment which is detrimental rather than the type of initial surgery used. Younger patients with good prognosis stage I disease (stage Ia, grade 1 or 2, serous histology) do not necessarily require radical surgery and adjuvant chemotherapy. However, in this group the staging must be accurate or the prognosis can be drastically altered (Sevelda *et al.*, 1990; Soper *et al.*, 1992). An appropriate gynecological oncology opinion should be sought urgently because of the reliance on accurate staging. A suitably trained gynecological surgeon will be able to perform the staging with a minimum of morbidity (Mayer *et al.*, 1992) and the cytoreductive surgery with a better result (Eisenkop *et al.*, 1992) and the woman will then have her follow-up in a cancer center with its added survival advantages (Junor *et al.*, 1994). Whether this surgical staging should be done as an open procedure, as currently accepted, or via the laparoscope (Querleu and Leblanc, 1994) will be the center of the next debate. Audit of adnexal mass and ovarian cancer surgery performed using minimal access techniques is important in order to clarify whether laparoscopic surgery in this condition is indeed an advance.

Approximately 70% of cases of epithelial ovarian cancer present in an advanced nature. The present initial management of these women is by laparotomy. At this operation, the cancer is diagnosed and histological confirmation is obtained. The staging procedure is performed and the extent of disease is documented. The FIGO stage is an important independent prognostic indicator. At present, cytoreductive surgery is then performed as the first therapeutic maneuver before systemic chemotherapy is given. This surgery aims to remove the bulk of the tumor, leaving either no residual or deposits measuring less than 1–2 cm diameter. This is possible in over half of the patients presenting to a gynecological oncologist. There is a survival advantage in those women where there is complete tumor clearance. The role of laparoscopic surgery in these cases is usually limited. However, it can be used efficiently to diagnose and stage women with advanced cancer.

Care must be taken when introducing the first port as bowel may be stuck to the anterior abdominal wall. The use of the left upper quadrant for the insertion of a small diameter laparoscope can be helpful in these circumstances (Childers *et al.*, 1993b). Once the site and extent of adhesions have been determined, a midline port can be placed under direct vision, allowing the use of the camera

and 10 mm scope as usual. Clear views of the subdiaphragmatic areas are obtained with laparoscopy and multiple biopsies can be taken. The extent of cytoreductive surgery is by necessity limited using the laparoscopic approach. Some exponents suggest a subtotal hysterectomy. This is achieved by ligating or stapling the infundibulopelvic ligaments and then securing the uterine pedicles. A ligature is placed around the isthmus and tightened. The fundus of the uterus is removed with heavy hooked scissors. Diathermy is used to secure hemostasis. The uterine specimen is removed by morcellation. In our view, this represents poor surgical technique. The use of a subtotal hysterectomy is unnecessary. If primary chemotherapy is to be used or the disease is felt to inoperable, a D&C should be performed to assess the spread of the tumor into the uterine cavity and to exclude a coincidental endometrial primary cancer.

A problem encountered with laparoscopy and advanced ovarian cancer is the development of port site implantation. This has occurred on several occasions in our unit although Childers *et al.* (1994) reported an incidence of less than 1%. It may be related to the seepage of ascites through the port site. This implantation problem may be overcome by starting chemotherapy within 48 hours of the laparoscopy rather than the delay of 2–4 weeks seen in the usual medical oncology referrals.

Laparoscopy allows excellent views of the diaphragm and pelvis for staging for advanced disease and allows adequate directed biopsy for a histological diagnosis. However, it does not allow scope for adequate cytoreductive surgery. Its role may be the appropriate assessment of a woman with advanced ovarian cancer who can then be referred to a specialist unit for consideration of surgery and chemotherapy.

OTHER CANCERS

Operative laparoscopy can be useful in aiding diagnosis of women with unidentified carcinomatosis. Modification of other operations used in oncology to suit a laparoscopic approach is illustrated by reports about laparoscopic oophoropexy prior to radiation therapy. Letterie (1995) reports a technique for attaching the ovaries to the lateral peritoneum using a suturing technique prior to pelvic radiation. Clough *et al.* (1996) report a series of unilateral right oophoropexy prior to pelvic radiation. We have used laparoscopic staples to fix the ovaries in the pouch of Douglas below the uterosacral ligaments prior to radiation for lymphoma.

CONCLUSION

The use of advanced laparoscopy in gynecological oncology may be an important advance in some of the diseases which we manage. However, we must be sure that the women are offered the best and most successful treatment available rather than the latest fashion and careful audit of these laparoscopic procedures over the coming years will determine whether this surgery is indeed a step forward. This surgery should be carried out by trained gynecological oncology surgeons in suitable oncology units and not by general endoscopists, however, skillful. Not only is the surgical expertise, both at open and laparoscopic surgery, important but so is an overall understanding of the natural history of the disease process in the light of current non-surgical developments.

REFERENCES

Artman, R.E., Hoskins, W.J. and Bybrowe, M.C. (1987) Radical lymphadenectomy and pelvic lymphadenectomy for stage 1b carcinoma of the cervix: 21 years experience. *Gynecol Oncol*, **28**, 8–13.

Barton, D.P., Cavanagh, D., Roberts, W.S. *et al.* (1992) Radical hysterectomy for treatment of cervical cancer: a prospective study of two methods of closed-suction drainage. *Am J Obstet Gynecol*, **166**, 533–7.

Bjornsson, B.L., Nelson, B.E., Reale, F.R. and Rose, P.G. (1993) Accuracy of frozen section for lymph node metastasis in patients undergoing radical hysterectomy for carcinoma of the cervix. *Gynecol Oncol*, **51**, 50–3.

Bloss, J.D., Berman, M.L., Mukhererjee, J. *et al.* (1992) Bulky stage Ib cervical carcinoma managed by primary radical hysterectomy followed by tailored radiotherapy. *Gynecol Oncol*, **47**, 21–7.

Burghardt, E., Pickle, H., Haas, J. *et al.* (1987) Prognostic factors and operative treatment of stages 1b to 2b cervical cancer. *Am J Obstet Gynecol*, **156**, 988–96.

Canis, M., Mage, G., Pouly, J.L. *et al.* (1994) Laparoscopic diagnosis of adnexal cystic masses: a 12-year experience with long term follow-up. *Obstet Gynecol*, **83**, 707–12.

Childers, J.M., Hatch, K. and Surwit, E.A. (1992) The role of laparoscopic lymphadenectomy in the management of cervical cancer. *Gynecol Oncol*, **47**, 38–43.

Childers, J.M., Brzechffa, P.R., Hatch, K.D. and Surwitt, E.A. (1993a) Laparoscopically assisted surgical staging (LASS) of endometrial cancer. *Gynecol Oncol*, **51**, 33–8.

Childers, J.M., Brzechffa, P.R. and Surwit, E.A. (1993b) Laparoscopy using the left upper quadrant as the primary trocar site. *Gynecol Oncol*, **50**, 221–5.

Childers, J.M., Aqua, K.A., Surwit, E.A. *et al.* (1994) Abdominal-wall tumor implantation after laparoscopy for malignant conditions. *Obstet Gynecol*, **84**, 765–9.

Childers, J., Surwit, E., Hallum, A. and Hatch, K. (1995) Laparoscopic staging of ovarian cancer. *Gynecol Oncol*, **56**, 139.

Childers, J.M., Nassen, A. and Surwit, E.A. (1996) Laparoscopic management of suspicious adnexal masses. *Am J Obstet Gynecol*, **175**, 1451–9.

Cirocco, W.C., Schwartzman, A. and Golub, R.W. (1994) Abdominal wall recurrence after laparoscopic colectomy for colon cancer. *Surgery*, **116**, 842–6.

Clough, K.B., Goffinet, F., Labib, A. *et al.* (1996) Laparoscopic unilateral ovarian transposition prior to irradiation. *Cancer*, **77**, 2638–45.

Crawford, R.A.F., Richards, P.J., Reznek, R.H. *et al.* (1996) The role of CT in predicting the surgical feasibility of exenteratio in recurrent carcinoma of the cervix. *Int J Gynecol Cancer*, **6**, 231–4.

Crawford, R.A.F., Gore, M. and Shepherd, J.H. (1995) Ovarian cancers related to minimal access surgery. *Br J Obstet Gynaecol*, **102**, 726–30.

Creaseman, W.T., Morrow, C.P., Bundy, B.N. *et al.* (1987) Surgical pathologic spread patterns of endometrial cancer. *Cancer*, **60**(suppl), 2035–41.

Dargent, D., Brun, J.L., Roy, M. *et al.* (1994) La Trachélectomie élargie. *JOBGYN*, **2**, 285–92.

Davies, A.P., Jacobs, I., Woolas, R. *et al.* (1993) The adnexal mass: benign or malignant? Evaluation of a risk of malignancy index. *Br J Obstet Gynaecol*, **100**, 927–31.

Dembo, A.J., Davy, M., Stenwig, A.E. *et al.* (1990) Prognostic factors in patients with stage I epithelial ovarian cancer. *Obstet Gynecol*, **75**, 263–73.

Downey, G.O., Pottish, R.A., Adcock, L.L. *et al.* (1989) Pre-treatment surgical staging and cervical carcinoma: therapeutic efficacy of pelvic lymph node resections. *Am J Obstet Gynecol*, **160**, 1055–61.

Dressler, F. (1991) Zur endoskopischen Therapie von zystischen Ovarialtumouren und Paraovarialzysten. *Geburtsh u Frauenheilk*, **51**, 474–80.

Eisenkop, S.M., Spirtos, N.M., Montag, T.W. *et al.* (1992) The impact of subspeciality training on the management of advanced ovarian cancer. *Gynecol Oncol*, **147**, 203–9.

Faught, W., Krepart, G.V., Lotocki, R. and Heywood, M. (1994) Should selective paraaortic lymphadenectomy be part of surgical staging for endometrial cancer? *Gynecol Oncol*, **55**, 51–5.

Ferraris, G., Lanza, D'Addato, F. *et al.* (1988) Techniques of pelvic and para-aortic lymphadenectomy in the surgical treatment of cervix carcinoma. *Eur J Gynecol Oncol*, **9**, 83–6.

Fidalgo de Matos, C.J., Querleu, D. and Leblanc, E. (1993) La lymphadénectomie pelvienne endoscopique dans le bilan des cancers précoces du col utérin: enquête auprès de 35 centres hospitaliers français. *Rev Méd Brux*, **14**, 163–8.

Finn, C.B., Luesley, D.M., Buxton, E.J. *et al.* (1992) Is stage I epithelial ovarian cancer over treated both surgically and systemically? Results of a five year cancer registry review. *Br J Obstet Gynaecol*, **99**, 54–8.

Fowler, J.M., Carter, J.R., Carlson, J.W. *et al.* (1993) Lymph node yield from laparoscopic lymphadenectomy and cervical cancer: a comparative study. *Gynecol Oncol*, **51**, 187–92.

Fowler, J.M., Hartenbach, E.M., Reynolds, H.T. *et al.* (1994) Pelvic adhesion formation after pelvic lymphadenectomy: comparison between transperitoneal laparoscopy and extraperitoneal laparotomy in a porcine model. *Gynecol Oncol*, **55**, 25–8.

Fox, H. (1993) Pathology of early malignant change in the ovary. *Int J Gynecol Path*, **12**, 153–5.

Herrmann, U., Locher, G. and Goldhirsch, A. (1987) Sonographic patterns of ovarian tumours: prediction of malignancy. *Obstet Gynecol*, **69**, 777–81.

Homesley, H.D. (1996) Management of endometrial cancer. *Am J Obstet Gynecol*, **174**, 529–34.

Homesley, H.D., Kadar, N., Barrett, R.J. and Lentz, S.S. (1992) Selective pelvic and periaortic lymphadenectomy does not increase morbidity in surgical staging of endometrial cancer. *Am J Obstet Gynecol*, **167**, 1225–30.

Hoskins, W.J. (1988) Prognostic factors with a risk of recurrence in stages 1b and 2a cervical cancer, in *Clinical Obstetrics and Gynaecology*, (eds. E. Burghardt and J.M. Monaghan), Baillière Tindall, London, pp. 817–28.

Hulka, J.F., Parker, W.H., Surrey, M.W. and Phillips, J.M. (1992) Management of ovarian masses: AAGL 1990 survey. *J Reprod Med*, **37**, 559–602.

Johnson, N. (1994) Laparoscopic versus conventional pelvic lymphadenectomy for gynaecological malignancy. *Br J Obstet Gynaecol*, **101**, 902–4.

Johnson, N., Johnson, V., McKie, G. and Knowles, S. (1994) Laparoscopic pelvic lymphadenectomy versus traditional surgery in pigs. *Br J Obstet Gynaecol*, **101**, 901–2.

Junor, E.J., Hole, D.J. and Gillis, C.R. (1994) Management of ovarian cancer: referral to a multidisciplinary team matters. *Br J Cancer*, **70**, 363–70.

Kavoussi, L., Sosa, E., Chandhoke, P. *et al.* (1993) Complications of laparoscopic pelvic lymph node dissection. *J Urol*, **149**, 322–5.

Kerlikowske, K., Brown, J.S. and Grady, D.G. (1992) Should women with familial ovarian cancer undergo prophylactic oophorectomy? *Obstet Gynecol*, **80**, 700–7.

Kindermann, G., Maassen, V. and Kuhn, W. (1995) Laparoskopisches 'Anoperieren' von ovariellen Malignomen – Erfahrungen aus 127 deutschen Frauenkliniken. *Geburtsh u Frauenheilk*, **55**, 687–94.

Kottmaier, H.L. (ed.) (1982) Annual report on the results of treatment in gynaecologic cancer. *Int J Gynecol Obstet*, **18**.

Lees, D.H. (1978) The surgery of endometrial carcinoma. *Clinics Obstet Gynaecol*, **5**, 675–94.

Lehmann-Willenbrock, E., Mecke, H. and Semm, K. (1991) Pelviskopische Ovarialchirurgie – eine retrospektive Untersuchung von 1016 operierten Zysten. *Geburtsh u Frauenheilk*, **51**, 280–7.

Letterie, G.S. (1995) A laparoscopic technique for lateral oophoropexy to conserve ovarian function prior to abdominopelvic irradiation. *Surg Endosc*, **9**, 1144–5.

Levine, R.L. (1990) Pelviscopic surgery in women over 40. *J Reprod Med*, **35**, 597–600.

Liu, C.Y. (1992) Laparoscopic hysterectomy. *J Reprod Med*, **37**, 351–4.

Mage, G., Canis, M., Wattiez, A. *et al.* (1990) Hystérectomie et coeliscopie. *J Gynecol Obstet Biol Reprod*, **19**, 569.

Maiman, M., Seltzer, V. and Boyce, J. (1991) Laparoscopic excision of ovarian neoplasms subsequently found to be malignant. *Obstet Gynecol*, **77**, 563–5.

Massi, G., Savino, L. and Susini, T. (1996) Vaginal hysterectomy versus abdominal hysterectomy for treatment of stage 1 endometrial adenocarcinoma. *Am J Obstet Gynecol*, **174**, 1320–6.

Mayer, A.R., Chambers, S.K., Graves, E. *et al.* (1992) Ovarian cancer staging: does it require a gynecologic oncologist? *Gynecol Oncol*, **47**, 223–7.

Morris, P.C., Haugen, J., Anderson, B. and Buller, R. (1992) The significance of peritoneal cytology in stage Ib cervical cancer. *Obstet Gynecol*, **80**, 196–8.

Morrow, C.P. (1980) Panel report: is pelvic radiation beneficial in the post-operative management of stage 1b squamous cell carcinoma of the cervix with pelvic node metastases treated by radical hysterectomy and pelvic lymphadenectomy? *Gynecol Oncol*, **10**, 105–10.

Nahhas, W.A., Whitney, C.W., Stryker, J.A. *et al.* (1980) Stage II endometrial carcinoma. *Gynecol Oncol*, **10**, 303–11.

Nezhat, C., Winter, W. and Nezhat, F. (1989) Laparoscopic removal of dermoid cysts. *Obstet Gynecol*, **73**, 278–80.

Nezhat, F., Nezhat, C., Welander, C.E. and Benigno, B. (1992) Four ovarian cancers diagnosed during laparoscopic management of 1011 women with adnexal masses. *Am J Obstet Gynecol*, **167**, 790–6.

Nicklin, J.L., van Eijkeren, M., Athanasatos, P. *et al.* (1994) A comparison of ovarian cyst aspirate cytology and histology. The case against aspiration of cystic pelvic masses. *Aust NZ J Obstet Gynaecol*, **34**, 546–9.

Nilbert, M., Pejovic, T., Mandahl, N. *et al.* (1995) Monoclonal origin of endometriotic cysts. *Int J Gynecol Cancer*, **5**, 61–3.

Oram, D.H. (1990) The management of cancer of the uterine corpus, in *Clinical Gynaecological Oncology*, 2nd edn, (eds. J.H. Shepherd and J.M. Monaghan), Blackwell Scientific, Oxford, pp. 115–39.

Oram, D.H. and Bridges, J. (1987) Para-aortic lymphadenectomy. *Baillière's Clinical Obstetrics and Gynaecology*, **1**, 369–81.

Parker, W.H. (1992) Management of adnexal masses by operative laparoscopy: selection criteria. *J Reprod Med*, **37**, 603–6.

Parker, W.H. and Berek, J.S. (1990) Management of selected cystic adnexal masses by operative laparoscopy: a pilot study. *Am J Obstet Gynecol*, **163**, 1574–7.

Parker, W.H. and Berek, J.S. (1993) Management of adnexal mass by operative laparoscopy. *Clin Obstet Gynecol*, **36**, 413–22.

Patsner, B., Sedlacek, T.V. and Lovecchio, J.L. (1992) Para-aortic node sampling in small (3 cm or less) stage Ib invasive cervical cancer. *Gynecol Oncol*, **44**, 53–4.

Peters, W.A., Anderson, W.A., Thornton, W.N. and Morley, G.W. (1983) The selective use of vaginal hysterectomy in the management of adenocarcinoma of the endometrium. *Am J Obstet Gynecol*, **146**, 285–9.

Peterson, H., Hulka, J. and Phillips, J. (1990) American Association of Gynecologic Laparoscopists 1988 membership survey on operative laparoscopy. *J Reprod Med*, **35**, 587–9.

Plante, M. and Roy, M. (1995) The use of operative laparoscopy in determining eligibility for pelvic exenteration in patients with recurrent cervical cancer. *Gynecol Oncol*, **59**, 401–4.

Potter, M.E., Abrovez, R.D., Shingleton, H.M. *et al.* (1990) Early invasive cervical cancer with pelvic lymph node involvement: to complete or not to complete radical hysterectomy? *Gynecol Oncol*, **37**, 78–81.

Querleu, D. (1993) Laparoscopic para-aortic node sampling: preliminary experience. *Gynecol Oncol*, **49**, 24–9.

Querleu, D. and LeBlanc, E. (1994) Laparoscopic infrarenal paraaortic lymph node dissection for restaging of carcinoma of the ovary or fallopian tube. *Cancer*, **73**, 1467–71.

Querleu, D., LeBlanc, E. and Castelain, B. (1991) Laparoscopic pelvic lymphadenectomy in the staging of early carcinoma of the cervix. *Am J Obstet Gynecol*, **164**, 579–81.

RCOG (1994) *Report of the RCOG Working Party on Training in Gynaecological Endoscopic Surgery*, RCOG Press, London, p. 12.

Reich, H. (1987) Laparoscopic oophorectomy and salpingo-oophorectomy in the treatment of benign tubo-ovarian disease. *Int J Fertil*, **32**, 233.

Reich, H., Decaprio, J. and McGlynn, F. (1989) Laparoscopic hysterectomy. *J Gynecol Surg*, **5**, 213–16.

Reich, H., McGlynn, F. and Wilkie, W. (1990) Laparoscopic management of stage I ovarian cancer: a case report. *J Reprod Med*, **35**, 601–5.

Remy, J.C., di Maio, T., Fruchter, R.G. *et al.* (1990) Adjunctive radiation after radical hysterectomy in stage Ib squamous cell carcinoma of the cervix. *Gynecol Oncol*, **38**, 161–5.

Sainz de la Cuesta, R., Goff, B.A., Fuller, A.F. *et al.* (1994) Prognostic importance of intraoperative rupture of malignant ovarian epithelial neoplasms. *Obstet Gynecol*, **84**, 1–7.

Sedlacek, T.V., Campion, M.J., Reich, H. and Sedlacek, T. (1995) Laparoscopic radical hysterectomy: a feasibility study. *Gynecol Oncol*, **56**, 126.

Seltzer, V. (1993) Laparoscopic surgery for ovarian lesions: potential pitfalls. *Clin Obstet Gynecol*, **36**, 403–12.

Sevelda, P., Dittrich, C. and Salzer, H. (1989) Prognostic value of the rupture of the capsule in stage I epithelial ovarian carcinoma. *Gynecol Oncol*, **35**, 321–2.

Sevelda, P., Vavara, N., Schemper, M. and Salzer, H. (1990) Prognostic factors for survival in stage I epithelial ovarian carcinoma. *Cancer*, **65**, 2349–52.

Shepherd, J.H. (1989) Revised FIGO staging for gynaecological cancer. *Br J Obstet Gynaecol*, **96**, 889–992.

Shepherd, J.H. (1990) Surgical management of ovarian cancer, in *Clinical Gynaecological Oncology*, (eds. J.H. Shepherd and J.M. Monaghan), Blackwell Scientific, London, pp. 224–5.

Shepherd, J.H., Carter, P.G. and Lowe, D.G. (1994) Wound recurrence by implantation of a borderline ovarian tumor following laparoscopic removal. *Br J Obstet Gynaecol*, **101**, 265–6.

Sjövall, K., Nilsson, B. and Einhorn, N. (1994) Different types of rupture of the tumor capsule and the impact on survival in early ovarian carcinoma. *Int J Gynecol Cancer*, **4**, 333–6.

Soper, J.T., Johnson, P., Johnson, V. *et al.* (1992) Comprehensive restaging laparotomy in women with apparent early ovarian carcinoma. *Obstet Gynecol*, **80**, 949–53.

Spirtos, N.M., Schlaerth, J.B., Spirtos, T.W. *et al.* (1995) Laparoscopic bilateral pelvic and para-aortic lymph node sampling: an evolving technique. *Am J Obstet Gynecol*, **173**, 105–11.

Stellato, G., Tikkala, L., Makela, P. and Kajanoja, P. (1992) Pelvic lymph node metastases in cervical cancer: comparison of lymphangiography, inspection radiography and histologic examination of lymph nodes. *Europ J Gynecol Oncol*, **13**, 161–6.

Vergote, I.B., Kærn, J., Abeler, V.M. *et al.* (1993) Analysis of prognostic factors in stage I epithelial ovarian carcinoma: importance of degree of differentiation and deoxyribonucleic acid ploidy in predicting relapse. *Am J Obstet Gynecol*, **169**, 40–52.

Webb, M.J., Decker, D.G., Mussey, E. and Williams, T.J. (1973) Factors in influencing survival in stage I ovarian cancer. *Am J Obstet Gynecol*, **116**, 222–8.

Winter, R., Petru, E. and Haas, J. (1988) Pelvic and para-aortic lymphadenectomy in cervical carcinoma. *Baillières Clinical Obstetrics and Gynaecology*, **2**, 857–66.

A. Pooley

INTRODUCTION

During the last 20 years the use of laparoscopy by gynecologists has progressed from diagnosis and simple procedures such as sterilization, ventrosuspension and ovarian cyst aspiration to a situation where many of the classic major gynecological operations can be performed laparoscopically, including some procedures for pelvic malignancy. Many of these operations generate quite large volumes of tissue requiring removal.

Early methods of laparoscopic tissue removal, involving significant enlargement of an abdominal port or a large posterior colpotomy incision, seemed to negate the rationale for minimal access surgery, i.e. smaller less painful wounds with more rapid recovery. However, in the absence of specific extraction techniques, removing a large piece of tissue from the abdomen can be the most time-consuming and frustrating part of the operation. Before describing specific techniques, it is worthwhile discussing the areas in which problems may arise.

POTENTIAL PROBLEMS WITH TISSUE EXTRACTION

INCISIONAL HERNIA

Despite the small size of incisions used in operative laparoscopy, herniation of bowel or omentum has been reported (Kadar *et al.*, 1993), more commonly with laterally placed ports (Kurtz *et al.*, 1993; Patterson *et al.*, 1993).

COMPLICATIONS OF POSTERIOR COLPOTOMY

This route allows moderately large pieces of tissue to be removed, but the potential for infection, dyspareunia, adhesions, granulation tissue formation and rectal or ureteric injury exists.

INCOMPLETE REMOVAL OR SPILLAGE OF TISSUE

Ectopic pregnancy

The commonest problem encountered after conservative laparoscopic treatment of an ectopic pregnancy has been residual trophoblast within the tube, occurring in 5% of cases (Donnez and Nisolle, 1989), rising to 16% in cases of laparoscopic tubal milking (Chapron *et al.*, 1991).

Appendicitis

During laparoscopic appendicectomy the transection margin may contaminate the abdomen with fecal material if not isolated carefully.

Gynecological Endoscopic Surgery. Edited by C.J.G. Sutton. Published in 1997 by Chapman & Hall, London. ISBN 0 412 58040 3.

Ovarian tumors

Benign tumors

Intraoperative spillage of the contents of a mucinous cystadenoma may theoretically initiate pseudomyxoma peritonei, though the risk appears to be small (Mage *et al.*, 1990).

Teratomas

Chemical peritonitis and granuloma formation with intestinal obstruction has been reported after laparoscopic management of benign cystic teratomas (Langebrekke and Urnes, 1994). In this case, however, the entire capsules of bilateral cystic tumors were not removed and several series of laparoscopically managed teratomas exist without this complication (Mage *et al.*, 1990; Ulrich *et al.*, 1994).

Borderline and malignant tumors

Debate continues as to the dangers of spillage of the contents of borderline and malignant ovarian cysts, with some authors showing no change in prognosis (Grogan, 1967; Sigurdsson *et al.*, 1983) while others suggest spillage to be an important negative prognostic factor (Malkasian *et al.*, 1984).

CONTAMINATION OF THE PORT SITE

Simply pulling a specimen through an abdominal port has been reported to lead to implantation in the abdominal wall of both endometriosis (Sutton, 1993) and papillary serous carcinomas of the ovary (Hsiu *et al.*, 1986).

PROBLEMS WITH HISTOLOGICAL EXAMINATION OF SPECIMENS

Vaginal squames may contaminate an ovary pulled through a posterior colpotomy, confusing accurate histology. Morcellation, whilst not preventing histological examination of a specimen, will destroy surgical tissue margins (Clayman *et al.*, 1991) and make orientation more difficult for the pathologist.

MISPLACEMENT OF SPECIMENS IN THE ABDOMEN

A specimen placed on or allowed to fall onto the loops of bowel in the central abdomen at laparoscopy may sink without trace. One would hope to find the specimen in the pouch of Douglas at a later laparoscopy, but the need for a laparotomy to retrieve a transected uterus from beneath the spleen has been described (Semm, 1993).

PRACTICAL ASPECTS OF TISSUE EXTRACTION

Two criteria will dictate the methods suitable for removal: firstly, the size or volume of the specimen and secondly, depending on the likely pathology, the need to isolate the specimen within a retrieval device to avoid contamination during removal. If extraction is to be delayed, parking the specimen in the uterovesical pouch or the pouch of Douglas, in a laparoscopic gag, or against the abdominal wall with a suture is advisable.

SMALL SPECIMENS

The largest diameter to which a laparoscopic port can be enlarged before it becomes a minilaparotomy is probably about 20 mm. This can be done with a knife or with a specific port-enlarging device. These port enlargers are specifically designed to enlarge the umbilical incision to facilitate the removal of the gall bladder at laparoscopic cholecystectomy. On no account should they be used to enlarge lateral incisions because of the very real risk of tearing the inferior epigastric vessels which have been so carefully avoided during initial placement of the lower quadrant ports. The simplest method of removal is to grasp the tissue with a strong toothed grasping forceps

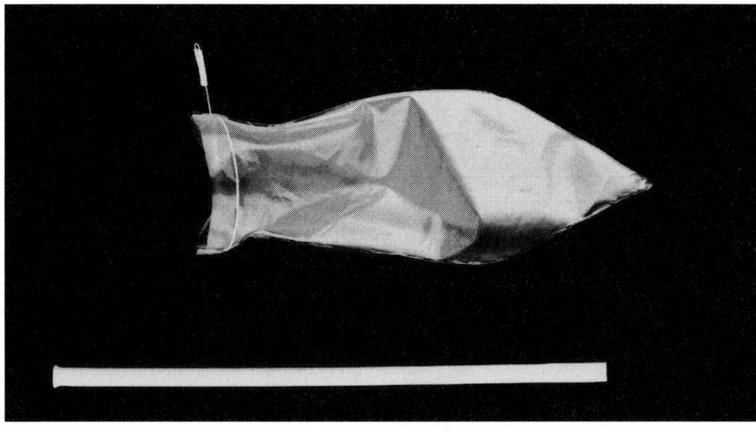

Figure 9.1   The Extraction Bag (Storz, Tuttlingen, Germany).

and pull it up the port cannula and through the valve. Some valves will allow tissue to be pulled through them. If this is not possible the trocar should be used with a screw-locking anchor which can be left *in situ* with a thumb over the end when the trocar containing the specimen is removed, to prevent loss of pneumoperitoneum. If plastic locking devices are used with monopolar electrosurgical instruments, great care must be taken. Capacitative coupling can occur if a hybrid port is created, in which the plastic locking anchor prevents dispersal of radio-frequency energy through the abdominal wall.

Several devices exist which allow isolation of a specimen. Olympus Keymed (Southend-on-Sea, UK) make 5, 15 and 20 mm diameter simple guiding tubes into which a specimen can be drawn and a 20 mm diameter extractor which seals the specimen in its shaft. Alternatively, a bag or sac can be used, examples of which include the Extraction Bag (Storz, Tuttlingen, Germany) (Figure 9.1), the Lapsac (Cook (UK), Letchworth; Cook Ob-Gyn, Spencer, USA) (Figure 9.2), the Pleatman Sac (Cabot Medical, Langhorne, USA) and the Endocatch (Autosuture, Ascot, UK; US Surgical Corporation, Norwalk, USA). With a range of sizes, all of these will allow isolation of a

specimen inside the abdomen. If the specimen is sufficiently small and malleable, the bag can be drawn through the port or through the abdominal wall after removing the port. Suitable specimens would be an ectopic pregnancy or a salpingectomy, an appendix, an endometrioma or its capsule or an ovary of normal size of uncertain pathology.

A novel method of removing salpingectomy specimens has been reported using commercially available condoms that have been washed in an antiseptic solution to remove the lubricant and spermicide (Trujillo *et al.*, 1994). Whilst costing little, potential risks of this technique include questionable asepsis, latex anaphylaxis (Swartz *et al.*, 1990) and splitting and fragmentation of the condom.

LARGER VOLUMES

With patience and ingenuity uterine fibroids up to 15 cm in diameter can be removed laparoscopically (Nezhat *et al.*, 1991). Other authors question the sense of time-consuming extraction of large specimens with prolonged anesthesia and operator fatigue (Daniell and Gurley, 1991). Specimens suitable for simple morcellation include uterine fibroids, subtotal hysterectomies and benign ovaries. It is worth

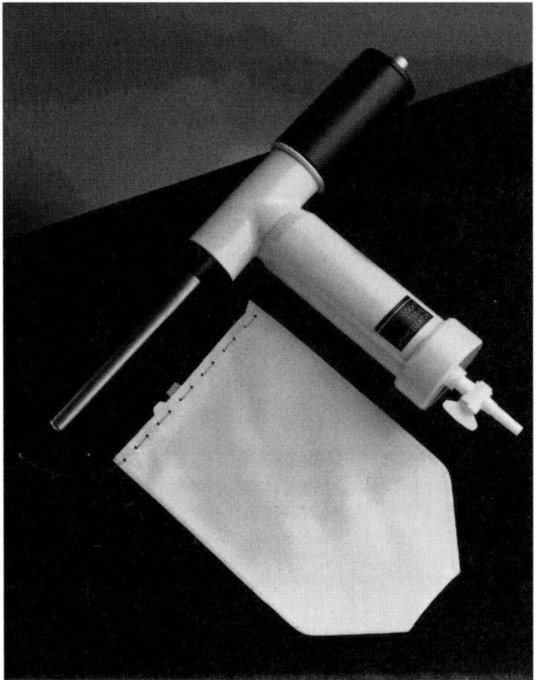

Figure 9.2 The Lapsac and Cook tissue morcellator (Cook (UK), Letchworth; Cook Ob-Gyn, Spencer, USA).

remembering that uterine fibroids can be reduced in volume by up to 40% using gonadotropin-releasing hormone analogs prior to surgery (Dubuisson *et al.*, 1992). In its simplests form morcellation can be achieved using graspers and endoscopic scissors, cutting diathermy or laser energy to yield pieces small enough to pull through a port. Alternatively the specimen can be pulled against an abdominal incision or posterior colpotomy through which a small knife is inserted to divide it. This technique can be difficult and potentially dangerous. Devices exist for both manual and mechanical morcellation.

The hand-operated tissue punch (Storz, Tuttlingen, Germany), first described in 1978 by Semm, takes bites of tissue which are pushed up the 11 mm diameter shaft of the instrument. It is said to be inadequate for large tissue volumes and unable to deal with firm or calcified specimens (Steiner *et al.*, 1993). Two devices are currently available which will mechanically morcellate large volumes of tissue.

The Cook tissue morcellator (Cook (UK), Letchworth) (Figure 9.2) was first described for the laparoscopic removal of a 190 g tumor-bearing kidney through an 11 mm port (Clayman *et al.*, 1991). The disposable morcellator is connected to a reusable power unit and a suction supply. The tissue for removal needs to be placed in an isolating bag the mouth of which is pulled through the abdominal wall. The cutting cannula is then placed into the bag. Using the foot switch the specimen is then morcellated and aspirated from within the bag.

The Steiner electromechanical morcellator (Storz, Tuttlingen, Germany) (Figure 9.3) was introduced in 1993 (Steiner *et al.*, 1993). This reusable device allows morcellation inside the abdomen under laparoscopic observation. The instrument has a motor-driven cutting tube 13 mm in diameter. After inserting the tube, claw forceps are passed down the shaft to grasp the specimen. Using a foot switch, the tube is then rotated whilst pulling the specimen against the mouth of the tube. Cylinders of tissue are cut which are pulled up the shaft and are suitable for histological examination. The speed and direction of rotation of the tube can be varied.

Large volumes of tissue which need isolation before removal can be placed within one of the larger laparoscopic bags. Suitable specimens would include ovarian teratomas and mucinous cysts and any ovary about which there is concern regarding neoplasia. Errors in laparoscopic assessment of ovarian cysts are well documented (Maiman *et al.*, 1991). Others have shown that with strict adherence to guidelines of preoperative ultrasound assessment and intraoperative inspection, laparoscopic management of adnexal cystic masses appears to be safe (Mage *et al.*, 1990). Indeed, the laparoscopic management of stage Ia and Ib ovarian carcinoma is now advocated by some (Reich *et al.*, 1990).

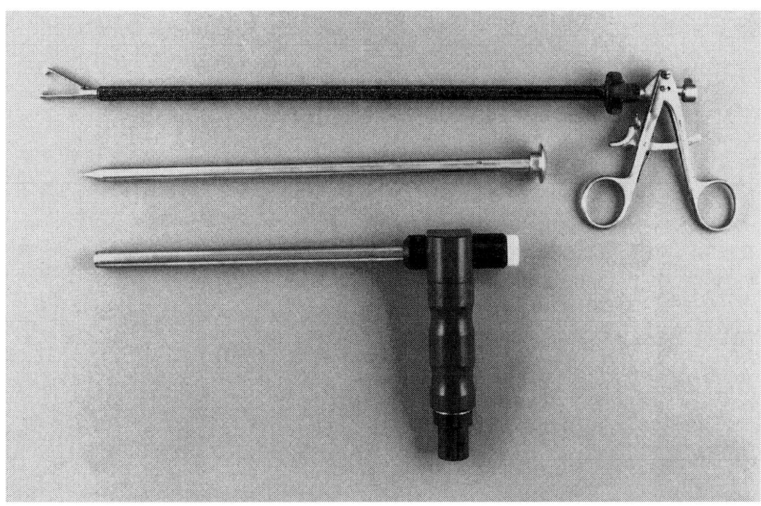

Figure 9.3   The Steiner electromechanical morcellator (Storz, Tuttlingen, Germany).

Once inside a bag cystic masses can be decompressed by incision and aspiration of their contents. This can be done inside the abdomen or after pulling the mouth of the bag outside the abdominal wall. Whilst malignant tumors can be safely removed using aspiration and morcellation with the mouth of the bag outside the abdomen (Clayman *et al.*, 1991), some authors are against this technique for suspicious masses, advocating intact extraction using a bag and an enlarged abdominal or colpotomy incision (Canis *et al.*, 1994).

With patience and ingenuity the specimens generated by operative laparoscopy can be removed without resorting to enlarged incisions. The use of such techniques for suspicious and malignant masses clearly needs long-term evaluation of large series before widespread acceptance can be anticipated.

REFERENCES

Canis, M., Mage, G., Wattiez, A. *et al.* (1994) The role of laparoscopic surgery in gynaecological oncology. *Current Opinion Obstet Gynecol*, **6**, 210–14.

Chapron, C., Querleu, D. and Crepin, G. (1991) Laparoscopic treatment of ectopic pregnancies. A one hundred cases study. *Eur J Obstet Gynaecol Reprod Biol*, **41**, 4–13.

Clayman, R., Kavoussi, L., Soper, N. *et al.* (1991) Laparoscopic nephrectomy: initial case report. *J Urol*, **146**, 278–82.

Daniell, J. and Gurley, L. (1991) Laparoscopic treatment of clinically significant symptomatic uterine fibroids. *J Gynecol Surg*, **7**, 37–40.

Donnez, J. and Nisolle, M. (1989) Laparoscopic treatment of ampullary tubal pregnancy. *J Gynecol Surg*, **5**, 157–62.

Dubuisson, J.B., Lecuru, F., Foulot, H. *et al.* (1992) Gonadotrophin-releasing hormone agonist and laparoscopic myomectomy. *Clin Therapeutics*, **14**(suppl), 51–6.

Grogan, R.H. (1967) Accidental rupture of malignant ovarian cysts during surgical removal. *Obstet Gynecol*, **30**, 716.

Hsiu, J., Given, F., Kemp, G. *et al.* (1986) Tumour implantation after diagnostic laparoscopic biopsy of serous ovarian tumours of low malignant potential. *Obstet Gynecol*, **3**(suppl), 90–3.

Kadar, N., Reich, H., Liu, C. *et al.* (1993) Incisional hernia after major laparoscopic gynaecological procedures. *Am J Obstet Gynecol*, **168**, 1493–5.

Kurtz, B.R., Daniell, J., Spaw, A. *et al.* (1993) Incarcerated incisional hernia after laparoscopy. A case report. *J Reprod Med*, **38**, 643–4.

Langebrekke, A. and Urnes, A. (1994) Postoperative

complications after laparoscopic removal of benign cystic teratoma. *Gynecol Endosc*, **3**, 245–6.

Mage, G., Canis, M., Manhes, H. *et al.* (1990) Laparoscopic management of adnexal cystic masses. *J Gynecol Surg*, **6**, 71–9.

Maiman, M., Seitzer, V., Boyce, J. *et al.* (1991) Laparoscopic excision of ovarian neoplasms subsequently found to be malignant. *Obstet Gynecol*, **77**, 563–5.

Malkasian, G.D., Meiton, L., O'Brien, P. *et al.* (1984) Prognostic significance of histologic classification and grading of epithelial malignancies of the ovary. *Am J Obstet Gynecol*, **149**, 274.

Nezhat, C. *et al.* (1991) Laparoscopic myomectomy. *Int J Fertil*, **36**, 275–80.

Patterson, M., Walters, D., Bravder, W. *et al.* (1993) Postoperative bowel obstruction following laparoscopic surgery. *Am Surgeon*, **59**, 656–7.

Reich, H., McGlynn, F. and Wilkie, W. (1990) Laparoscopic management of stage I ovarian carcinoma: a case report. *J Reprod Med*, **35**, 601–5.

Semm, K. (1978) Tissue-puncher and loop ligation – new aid for surgical therapeutic pelviscopy (laparoscopy) endoscopic intraabdominal surgery. *Endoscopy*, **10**, 119–24.

Semm, K. (1993) Hysterectomy by pelviscopy: an alternative approach without colpotomy, in *Laparoscopic Hysterectomy*, (eds. R. Garry and H. Reich), Blackwell Scientific, London, pp. 118–32.

Sigurdsson, K. *et al.* (1983) Prognostic factors in malignant ovarian tumours. *Gynecol Oncol*, **15**, 370.

Steiner, R. *et al.* (1993) Electrical cutting device for laparoscopic removal of tissue from the abdominal cavity. *Obstet Gynecol*, **81**, 471–4.

Sutton, C.J.G. (1993) A practical approach to diagnostic laparoscopy, in *Endoscopic Surgery For Gynaecologists*, (eds. C.J.G. Sutton and M. Diamond), W.B. Saunders, London, pp. 21–7.

Swartz, J., Braude, B., Gilmour, R. *et al.* (1990) Intraoperative anaphylaxis to latex. *Can J Anaesthet*, **37**, 589–92.

Trujillo, J., Molina, A. and Parache, J. (1994) Laparoscopic extraction of a tubal pregnancy using a condom. *Gynecol Endosc*, **3**, 241–3.

Ulrich, U., Keckstein, J. and Karageorgieva, E. (1994) Ovarian mature teratoma: technical aspects of laparoscopic removal. *Gynecol Endosc*, **3**, 169–72.

LASER TREATMENT OF MALIGNANT GYNECOLOGIC GROWTHS

R. Kurek and D. Wallwiener

INTRODUCTION

Laser intervention has now become well integrated into gynecology and the main field of laser utilization is gynecologic endoscopy. The most common lasers are the CO_2 and Nd-YAG laser. They are extremely precise cutting instruments, with a thermal tissue effect which helps to insure effective hemostasis (Frank, 1992). Lysis of adhesions (Bhatta *et al.*, 1993), ovariolysis (Daniell and Miller, 1989) and the treatment of tubal pregnancies with maintenance of the tubo-ovarian functional unit (Lavy *et al.*, 1987; Gast *et al.*, 1988) are all indications for laser intervention. A further special feature of the CO_2 laser is the vaporization of endometriosis implants (Gast *et al.*, 1988; Corson *et al.*, 1989).

Oncology is an important branch of gynecology and treatment is made up of the trio of surgery, radiotherapy and chemotherapy. From a clinical point of view oncological treatment has two different aims. The major aim of tumor treatment is curative in nature so early diagnosis is of paramount importance. Radiographic and sonographic images with a high resolution are used to improve diagnostic reliability. Molecular biological and genetic examination methods, which should enable optimum assessment of the risk entailed, are also becoming increasingly important. Treatment usually comprises organ maintenance (where possible), oncological surgery and radiotherapeutical procedures, as well as systemic chemotherapy and hormone treatment. Combination treatment is the main approach, e.g. intraoperative radiation treatment (IORT) and primary chemotherapy followed by radiation in breast-maintaining treatment of mammary carcinomas. If curative treatment is no longer possible, palliative measures must be undertaken.

Palliative treatment is a major field of clinical research. Such therapy is usually necessary for local recurrences and extensive metastatic spread. It is, furthermore, often the only alternative for high-risk inoperable patients with numerous concurrent diseases. It is thus, by its very nature, mainly indicated in older women.

Demographic development has led to an ever-increasing percentage of older patients needing palliative treatment. The aim of palliative research is thus to supplement the existing range of treatment in order to improve the quality of life and the dignity of these women.

Effective oncological laser treatment differs fundamentally from laser intervention in infertility surgery. The aim is no longer tissue separation with the minimum possible traumatization of the surrounding tissue, but rather the maximum destruction of the malignant area. Currently three procedures are being tested:

1. CO_2 laser vaporization;
2. laser-induced interstitial thermotherapy (LITT);
3. photodynamic therapy (PDT).

Gynecological Endoscopic Surgery. Edited by C.J.G. Sutton. Published in 1997 by Chapman & Hall, London. ISBN 0 412 58040 3.

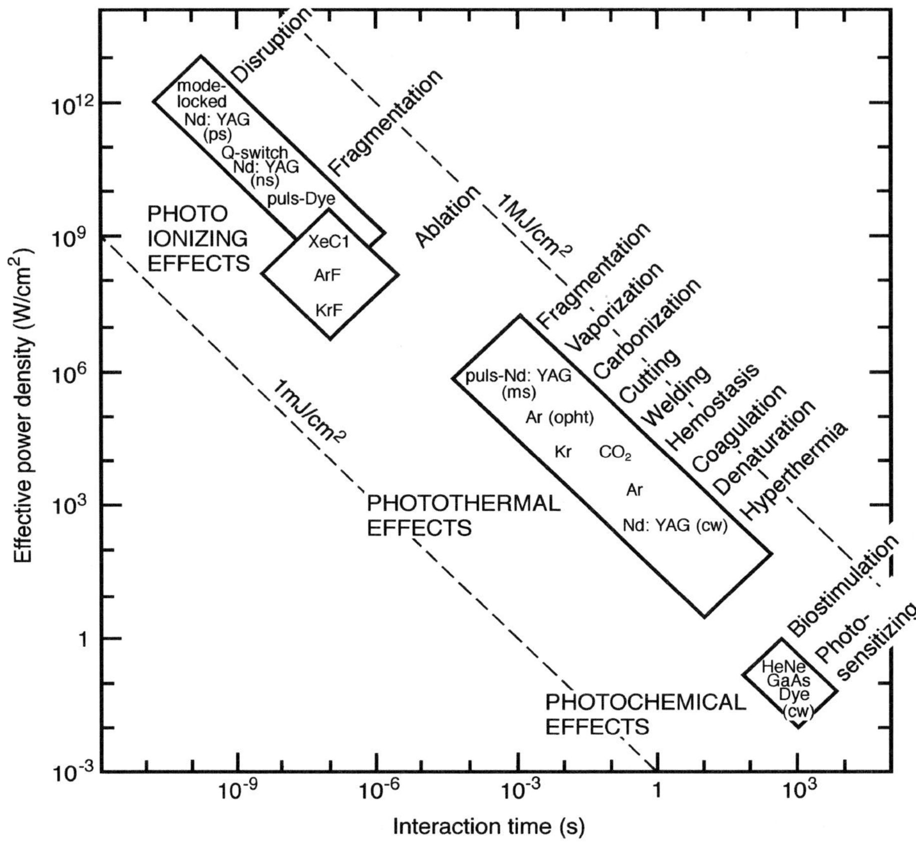

Figure 10.1   Photochemical, photothermal and photoionizing tissue effects of different laser therapeutical procedures.

These three methods all have different tissue effects and utilize different lasers (Figure 10.1). The aim of the treatment thus also varies.

CO_2 LASER VAPORIZATION

PHYSICAL FUNDAMENTALS AND BIOLOGICAL MECHANISMS

The CO_2 laser is the most common surgical laser, which usually has a mirror system integrated into an articulated arm. The light emitted from the resonator is transmitted to the operation site via this mirror system. It is not possible to transmit the laser beam effectively via flexible quartz glass fibers (Frank, 1992).

The laser beam is focused by a lens and can be enclosed in a handpiece or in an immobile endoscopic optical system. The latter is inserted in a trocar. Both single and double puncture techniques are possible during laparoscopic utilization of the CO_2 laser.

The CO_2 laser emits light with a wavelength of 10 600 nm. This light has its greatest absorption coefficient in water; a 1% extinction is obtained at a depth of 0.06 mm. Only a minimum of light quanta are scattered within the tissue (Frank, 1992). Human tissue is made up of a high percentage of water, hence almost the entire focused light energy is absorbed on the surface of the tissue and converted into thermal energy. A power density of less than

$100\,W/cm^2$ is easy to obtain (Hukki *et al.*, 1989). This results in instantaneous heating of the cellular and tissue fluid to over 100°C and thus in a rupture of the cellular membrane due to vaporization.

During thermal incision the CO_2 laser beam is focused on a minute point with a high power density, enabling a cutting action with almost no peripheral coagulation zones (Pogrel *et al.*, 1990), which develop because the distribution of the power output within the focused laser beam corresponds to a Gaussian distribution (Frank, 1992). The power density is lower at the edges of the laser beam and the energy there is too low for vaporization purposes; slight carbonization as well as minimal coagulation thus result (Lanzafame *et al.*, 1988). A second physical aspect which results in carbonization and coagulation is the exposure time. The surrounding tissue is heated when the threshold value is exceeded (Van Gemert and Welch, 1989). This can be avoided by only applying the maximum power density for fractions of a second (Walsh *et al.*, 1988). The advantage of utilizing the laser in the pulsed rather than the continuous wave (CW) mode is that higher power densities can be obtained, thus reducing the exposure time. Extremely high power densities can be attained for milliseconds by using the superpulsed mode with special pulsation methods (Lanzafame *et al.*, 1988). An ablative effect (i.e. vaporization without any residual components) results. A similar result can be obtained by very rapid transit of the laser beam over the target through the use of rapidly rotating mirrors (Swift Lase, Sharplan, Tel Aviv, Israel).

In contrast to cutting under maximum focus, oncological utilization of the CO_2 laser aims at the total destruction of a maximum volume of malignant tissue. In view of the high absorption coefficient one can speak of a maximum surface which should be vaporized. For this reason the laser beam must be defocused. There are two techniques available with which a power density (J/cm^2) great enough for vaporization purposes can be obtained:

1. lasers with an extremely high initial power output (which are, however, very expensive);
2. a focused laser beam, transmitted via a mechanical unit made up of two rotating mirrors, scans a round surface for fractions of a second, describing a geometric shape on this surface. During this maneuver every point on this surface is irradiated. The high speed with which the laser beam is transmitted through the rotating mirrors insures that the time-dependent thermal conduction is fully utilized.

EXPERIMENTAL AND CLINICAL UTILIZATION

Initial utilization of the CO_2 laser as a thermal scalpel showed that it has a number of advantages:

1. reduction in hemorrhage;
2. protection of the surrounding tissue;
3. reduction in postoperative pain;
4. less infection of the wound.

The possibility of using it for tumor resection thus seemed feasible.

During the first oncological studies on laser utilization, the laser was used as a thermal scalpel (Mahn *et al.*, 1982). The possible advantages of tumor resection by means of laser vaporization were investigated after it became evident that the laser was not ideal as a thermal scalpel after all. There is no mechanical traumatization during the laser extirpation of a malignant growth, hence the dissemination of tumor cells would probably be reduced. Experimental studies with animals (Peled *et al.*, 1976; Mahn *et al*; 1982; Sava *et al.*, 1982) examined the influence of laser vaporization on the long-term survival rate, local recurrences and metastatic spread. Our own study also investigated whether the type of energy applied, i.e. continuous wave, pulsed or superpulsed, influences the postoperative course (Wallwiener *et al.*, 1990). A Lewis lung carcinoma was implanted in mice and the tumor was excised six days later using different types of energy, the postoperative observations extending over 72 days. A further group of animals was treated with a steel scalpel and yet another group left untreated as a control group.

The postoperative survival time was longer in the laser groups than in the scalpel group. Furthermore, the local recurrence rate was reduced, as was pulmonary metastasis. These results are similar to those obtained by other study groups (Peled *et al.*, 1976; Mahn *et al.*, 1982; Sava *et al.*, 1982). The thermal effect within the wound bed results in the occlusion of small lymphatics and blood vessels, which may reduce the mechanical dissemination of vital tumor cells.

There was a distinct difference in the local recurrence rate within the laser groups, dependent upon the mode of application. The best results were obtained when the tumor bed was vaporized using the CW mode after the tumor had been removed (Wallwiener *et al.*, 1990).

There are serveral studies on the clinical utilization of the CO_2 laser to vaporize breast and ovarian carcinomas (Giebel and Jaeger, 1991; Fannin *et al.*, 1994).

After our experimental study we tested CO_2 laser vaporization for the palliative treatment of breast cancer in a clinical pilot study (Wallwiener *et al.*, 1991). The patients comprised two major groups:

1. women with generalized metastatic spread and advanced, often ulcerating soft tissue metastases;
2. women with local and regional recurrences which were inoperable due to their poor general condition.

On the basis of the results of our experimental study we combined CO_2 laser vaporization with subsequent deep coagulation of the wound bed using the Nd-YAG laser. This pilot study confirmed the advantages of laser utilization mentioned above. Furthermore, a positive psychological effect was observed. The possibility of carrying out the treatment under local anesthesia implied that it could be repeated without placing an unnecessary strain on the patients (Plate 3).

The study was extended to include metastases in general, including those located in the vulvovaginal area. Generally one can conclude that effective treatment of local and regional recurrences is only possible if the metastases are isolated, superficial and have a diameter <2 cm. No statements can be made concerning the metastatic dissemination rate because all the patients already had distant metastases when this purely palliative treatment was commenced.

Eisenkop *et al.* (1993) conducted an interesting study on the utilization of CO_2 laser vaporization for the treatment of ovarian carcinomas. They examined whether supplementary cytoreduction during surgical treatment of ovarian carcinomas increases the efficacy of subsequent chemotherapy and if the long-term survival rate is positively influenced. Once the abdomen had been opened tumor tissue was excised with a scalpel until there were no malignant tissue residues visible macroscopically. If it was not possible to remove the entire tumor with the scalpel, CO_2 laser vaporization was performed until there was no more malignant tissue discernible macroscopically. Adjuvant chemotherapy was administered postoperatively.

It is well known that maximum macroscopic resection of malignant growths increases the efficacy of adjuvant postoperative chemotherapy. In a retrospective study with 395 patients and a follow-up of 48 months, Wharton *et al.* (1984) were able to demonstrate that the survival time was 14% in the group with tumors >2 cm, whereas it increased to 40% in the group with tumors <2 cm. The patients observed by Eisenkop *et al.* included 67 women with ovarian carcinomas of the type FIGO-IIIc, the average follow-up extending over 46 months. The survival time was significantly increased in the patient group with supplementary cytoreduction compared to those in whom tumor implants <1 cm still remained after surgical intervention.

Eisenkop and colleagues also used the argon beam coagulator and ultrasound aspirator in addition to the CO_2 laser. The CO_2 laser has distinct advantages as far as handling is concerned:

1. the argon beam coagulator results in extensive carbonization which reduces the visibility and it must therefore be repeatedly removed (Eisenkop *et al.*, 1993);
2. the ultrasound aspirator works best in parenchymatous tissue due to its physical properties (Deppe *et al.*, 1988). Its effectiveness is thus highly tissue dependent, whereas the CO_2 laser vaporization effect is entirely independent of the type of tissue being treated.

CONCLUSION

The results of CO_2 laser vaporization of gynecologic malignant growths have shown this laser to be an effective instrument for the palliative treatment of multiple small metastases. The advantages this technique offers are controllable wound formation, reduction in postoperative pain and repeatability under local anesthesia.

The CO_2 laser is also effective for the removal of macroscopically visible tumor residues in a combination of surgical treatment of ovarian carcinomas with postoperative adjuvant chemotherapy. The efficacy of the adjuvant chemotherapy is thus enhanced. A major advantage is the removal of thin layers of tissue, as underlying structures are not endangered.

The most important limitation of the CO_2 laser is that it is not suitable for bulky tumors: its use is restricted to thin-layered, superficial tumors with a small diameter (<2 cm).

LASER-INDUCED INTERSTITIAL THERMOTHERAPY (LITT)

PHYSICAL FUNDAMENTALS AND BIOLOGICAL MECHANISMS

It is possible to coagulate tumor tissue with a diameter of several centimeters by means of laser-induced interstitial thermotherapy (LITT) (Masters *et al.*, 1992a; Muschter *et al.*, 1993; Wallwiener *et al.*, 1995a). LITT also functions according to the principle of the conversion of light quanta into thermal energy (Beuthan, 1992).

During LITT a special light guide is introduced into the center of the malignant tissue. The tissue is then irradiated for several minutes by laser light with a wavelength of 910–1064 nm. An almost ellipsoidal coagulation zone develops around the end of the fiber (Plate 4). The resulting thermal distention is dependent upon the selected laser parameters (initial laser output and irradiation time) as well as on the optical tissue parameters and the morphologically dependent thermal transmission properties of the tissue (Beuthan, 1992).

The initial laser output cited in the literature ranges from 2 to 7 watts, corresponding to a power density (dependent on the surface of the active zone of the light applicator) of 2–5 W/cm^2. The maximum irradiation time is usually quoted as 300–900 seconds (Beuthan, 1992; Masters *et al.*, 1992a; Muschter *et al.*, 1993; Wallwiener *et al.*, 1995a). Irradiation times longer than 1200 seconds do not result in a further distention of the thermally damaged area (Wallwiener *et al.*, 1994). Coagulation zones with a diameter of up to 3 cm can be attained.

LITT must not be confused with the hyperthermal techniques also utilized in oncological treatment. Hyperthermia is carried out at a temperature of only approximately 47°C, which does not lead to irreversible damage of the protein structures as a result of denaturation (Oleson *et al.*, 1993).

The mode of action of hyperthermia is thermal stress at a cellular level, which results in enzymatic and metabolic damage with cytotoxic consequences (Dewey, 1989). This procedure can be reversed, so there is no final damage, merely a certain percentage of the cells dying (Sapareto *et al.*, 1978; Borrelli *et al.*, 1990). In contrast, the denaturation process evident in the macroscopically visible coagulation necrosis induced by LITT is irreversible.

The main principle of LITT is the thermal conductivity of human tissue. Temperature determinations showed that the tissue immediately around the applicator achieves a temperature only marginally less than that of the vaporization range (Beuthan, 1992). There is a gradual decrease in temperature from the center of the coagulation zone to the edges (Figure 10.2). Coagulation commences at about 60°C, this being the temperature range of the edges. A narrow hyperemic edge surrounds the coagulation area of the *in vivo* specimen before normal tissue recommences. The morphological changes are discernible in histologic specimens: dilated, partially hyalinized vessels and alterations in the structure of collagenic bundles of fibers. The progression to normal tissue occurs without a clear demarcation.

Thermal conductivity is the major factor influencing the dimension of the thermally damaged zone and is more important than the optic tissue properties. Wyman *et al.* (1992) demonstrated this in their study. They compared the coagulation zones obtained with a bare laser fiber, a photo-optic source of energy and a fiber with the bare end covered with a metal cap, which thus functioned as a point source of energy. More extensive coagulation zones could be attained within a shorter period of time using the latter method. The extent of the damage caused by the bare fiber could be increased by increasing the temperature until the tissue began to carbonize. Carbonizing tissue fully absorbs the emitted radiation, thus the fiber henceforth only functions as a point source of thermal energy. Supporting proof of this can be found in the fact that the diode laser is comparable with the Nd-YAG laser although the absorption coeffi-

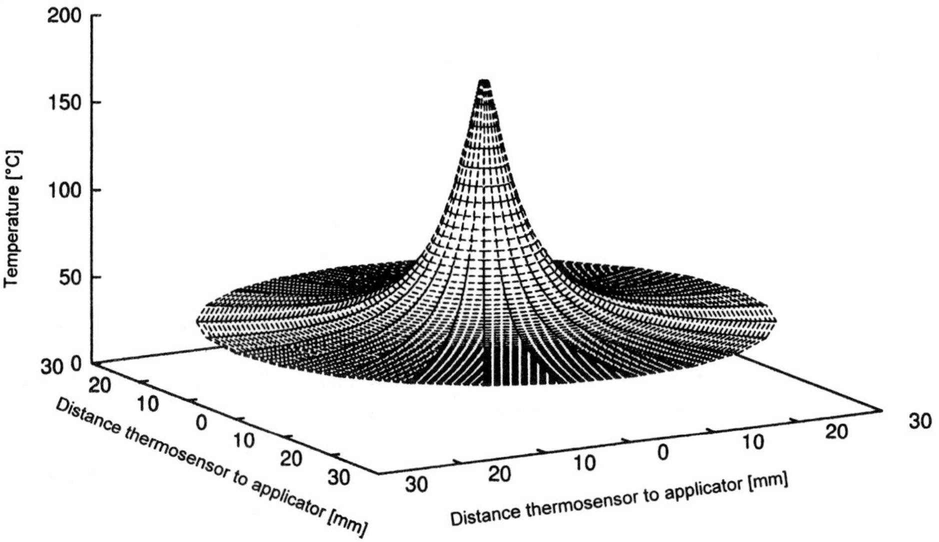

Figure 10.2 Monitoring of heat conduction in pig liver with a system of thermosensors at different distances from the LITT applicator (courtesy of M. Niemz PhD, Institute of Applied Physics, University of Heidelberg).

cient is three times as high at a wavelength of 810 nm (Jacques, 1992). One must bear in mind that the accumulated thermal energy can still cause further extension of the necrotic zone by heat conduction even minutes after the laser has been switched off.

The type of distention varies from tissue to tissue as does the extent of the necrosis. A regular distention in a rotation ellipsoid is observed in homogeneous tissue (e.g. liver). This is greater for the same laser parameters than in heterogeneous tissue (e.g. transversely striated muscle) in which the distention is irregular with tongue-shaped fringes. This also can be observed by sonographic monitoring (Wallwiener *et al.*, 1995b). Additional light guides, so-called multifiber systems, can be utilized to further increase the total distention of the thermal necrosis. A beam splitter is attached to the laser so that the light energy is transferred equally onto numerous fibers (Figure 10.3).

CLINICAL UTILIZATION OF LITT

LITT is still in the clinical test phase and there are reports of clinical oncological testing in neurosurgery (Wallwiener *et al.*, 1995b) and general surgery (Masters *et al.*, 1992b). In gynecology LITT is being tested for the palliative treatment of malignant growths by Masters *et al.* (1992b) as well as by our own group (Wallwiener *et al.*, 1994).

To date three patients with recurrent vaginal tumors have received palliative LITT at our center. They had all been pretreated surgically as well as radiologically and chemotherapeutically. When the LITT was administered they were primarily inoperable. They were aware of the experimental nature of the treatment and had given informed consent. The bare fiber was placed under sonographic control. The temperature was monitored with a thermal probe and, where possible, by manual examination. A noticeable reduction in the tumor volume could be observed postoperatively for a fortnight in all patients. This

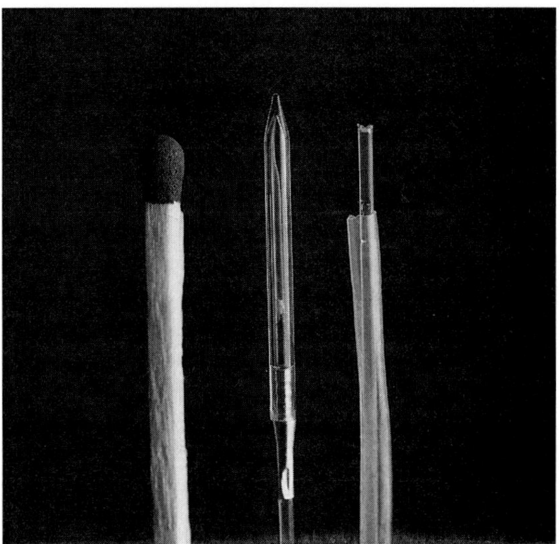

Figure 10.3 Applicator systems used for laser treatment. (*Left*) Conventional bare fiber; (*right*) LITT applicator.

corresponds with the results obtained in experimental studies (Anzai *et al.*, 1992). In one patient the residual tumor could be surgically removed after debulking by LITT.

Tissue examinations, experimental studies and clinical experience all show that LITT is well suited for the thermal destruction of solid tumors with a diameter of several centimeters. Muschter *et al.* (1994) showed that LITT is a gentle method of treating high-risk patients and ideal for the management of benign prostatic hyperplasia. He has treated the largest group of patients to date – 249. These included numerous high-risk patients who were treated under local anesthesia, as general anesthesia was not possible (Muschter *et al.*, 1993).

Currently the biggest problem in the therapeutic clinical utilization of LITT is that very few oncological patients have been treated with it to date. In contrast to the treatment of benign prostatic hyperplasia, which only aims at a shrinkage of the affected tissue, oncological utilization of LITT aims at the destruction of a maximum volume of malignant tissue without damaging the surrounding healthy tissue. This is all the more important as both neural and vascular structures can run directly next to a tumor. Furthermore, the extent of the thermally damaged zone is greatly influenced by the tissue morphology (Wallwiener *et al.*, 1995b) and the perfusion (Whelan and Wyman, 1995). An estimation of the thermal effect on the basis of laboratory findings is not justifiable. In an extensive tumor numerous bare fibers must be embedded (Stegner *et al.*, 1992) within it in a pattern in keeping with its shape. The additive coagulation effect between the applicators must, however, also be borne in mind.

PLANNING AND MONITORING OF LITT

Routine clinical utilization of LITT is governed by two prerequisites:

1. the existence of an effective on-line monitoring technique;
2. the use of a therapy simulation program enabling three-dimensional planning of the treatment with spatial tumor representation (CT, MRI) to ascertain both the ideal position of the fibers and the irradiation parameters.

Numerous tests have been undertaken to find possible ways of monitoring the treatment. There are two methods available:

1. ultrasonography (Masters *et al.*, 1992b; Stegner *et al.*, 1992) combined with Doppler flow measurements;
2. magnetic resonance imaging (MRI) (Castro *et al.*, 1990).

The coagulation necrosis can be sonographically represented on a B scan (Plate 5). The effectiveness is enhanced by combining it with Doppler flow measurements. Sonographic tumor representation is dependent upon the anatomic site of the tumor. Furthermore, an entire tumor cannot always be depicted on a single scan, hence this method can be problematic. Relevant for the accuracy of the B scan is the moment of image registration. Malone

and colleagues demonstrated in animal experiments that ultrasound showed too large a damage zone at the onset of laser coagulation and also that with increasing coagulation time, the coagulation zone is shown too small (Malone *et al.*, 1994).

The publications on sonographic monitoring (Castro *et al.*, 1990; Malone *et al.*, 1994; Wallwiener *et al.*, 1995b) also emphasize that tumor representation is highly dependent upon the type of equipment used as well as on the proficiency and experience of the ultrasonographic examiner.

Magnetic resonance imaging provides better possibilities of monitoring the temperature. MRI not only enables spatial representation of the thermal necrotic zone but also has the big advantage of temperature quantification. This thermal quantification is possible as MRI is capable of detecting diverse dimensions which are dependent upon the temperature. Possible parameters are the spin-grid-relaxation time T1 (Parker, 1993), the spin-spin-relaxation time T2 (Bottomley *et al.*, 1984; LeBihan *et al.*, 1989; Delannoy *et al.*, 1991), the molecular diffusion coefficient D of the tissue fluid and the chemical shift (Ishihara *et al.*, 1992; Lutz *et al.*, 1993). These methods are currently all still in the developmental phase.

The major problem often encountered with this method of monitoring LITT is the calculation time necessary for the generation of an image; this can take a few minutes, thus making simultaneous monitoring impossible. A solution to this problem does, however, appear to be in sight.

At present our team is carrying out a study in collaboration with the German Center for Cancer Research (DKFZ). We are testing a new method developed by the DKFZ which enables imaging within seconds (Stepanow *et al.*, 1993). Successful future MRI monitoring of LITT furthermore necessitates considerable infrastructural preconditions – the open MRI, which can be used intraoperatively. The first such instruments are currently being tested by neurosurgeons. MRI is also suited for postoperative surveillance of the thermal damage zone. Here the moment of image registration is important for accuracy of representation. Comparison of measurements of the coagulation zone on several days after the procedure by Tracz and coworkers (1993) showed that registration on the second day was the most accurate.

The only software available to date (Whiting, 1989; Miller, 1993; Roggan *et al.*, 1995) for the simulation of treatment was developed by the Laser Medical Center in Berlin (Roggan *et al.*, 1995). This program currently enables the two-dimensional simulation of a single bare fiber. A simulation program for the planning of LITT is based on calculations of the temperature distribution (Figure 10.4). Assessment models for LITT can be used (Davis *et al.*, 1989; Whiting, 1989; Miller, 1993), as well as models originating from research into hyperthermia (Lagendijk, 1987; Seebas *et al.*, 1983). The effect obtained by hyperthermia is differ-

ent, but the actual fundamental principle, i.e. thermal conduction, is the same as that of LITT.

There are currently no programs available which can be clinically utilized for three-dimensional temperature distribution. One of our future aims is thus to develop a three-dimensional temperature simulation program on the basis of a three-dimensional hyperthermia program and MRI measurements in collaboration with the DKFZ. The hyperthermia program (Seebas *et al.*, 1993) makes use of the method of finite element representation incorporated within three-dimensional CT and MRI data records.

CONCLUSION

Experience gathered to date has shown LITT to be potentially effective at destroying solid tumors. It thus compensates for the disadvantages inherent in CO_2 laser vaporization. Both

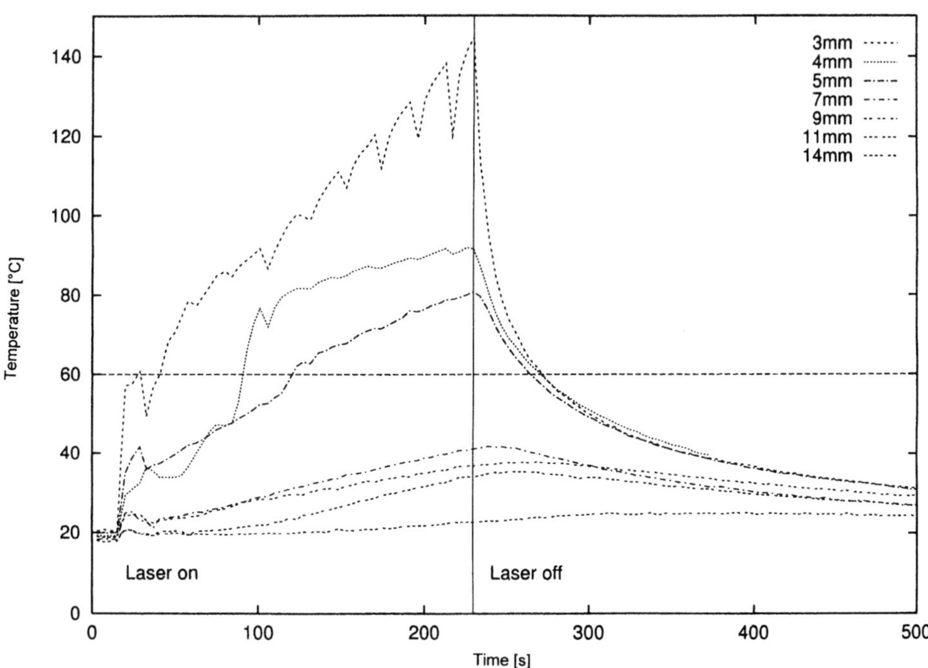

Figure 10.4 Simulation of heat distribution in liver tissue during LITT (courtesy of M. Niemz PhD, Institute of Applied Physics, University of Heidelberg).

methods are suitable for palliative treatment of high-risk patients who cannot undergo general anesthesia.

Before the clinical studies can be extended the current problems concerning the simulation and monitoring of LITT must first be overcome. This appears to be possible within the near future.

It will also be interesting to see if the less expensive alternatives to laser treatment, e.g. the monopolar high frequency technique, will be fully accepted. *In vitro* tests on a system comprising a monopolar HF generator and needle electrodes, which was specially developed for thermal treatment, showed this system to be superior to that of laser-induced interstitial thermotherapy (Wallwiener *et al.*, 1995a).

PHOTODYNAMIC THERAPY (PDT)

PHYSICAL AND CHEMICAL FUNDAMENTALS

Photodynamic therapy (PDT) is entirely different from the two methods of treatment discussed above, which both have a thermal mode of action. PDT, on the other hand, functions on the basis of the photochemical reaction which takes place when a particular substance – a photosensitizing agent (Figure 10.5) – administered before beginning the treatment, is activated by laser light. This reaction not only necessitates the simultaneous presence of both laser light and a photosensitizing agent, but also requires oxygen (Foote, 1990; Moan, 1992).

The molecules of the photosensitizing agent are electronically excited to a higher energy level, the triple excitation state, when struck by light quanta. There are numerous relaxation possibilities available to release this energy. Only two, however, are significant for PDT:

1. Photoreaction type I – the sensitizing agent reacts directly with the cell components, e.g. the cell membrane. Chemically reactive radicals and radical ions develop, which in turn are converted into oxygenated products by the reaction with oxygen (Fiel *et al.*, 1981).

2. Photoreaction type II – the excited

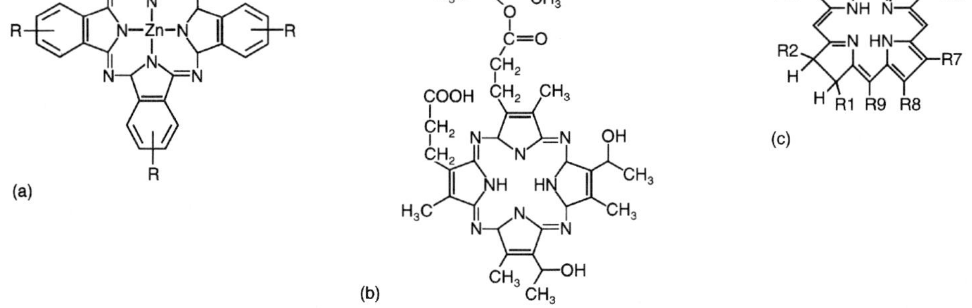

Figure 10.5   Chemical structures of different photosensitizers used for PDT. (a) Zinc phthalocyanine; (b) dihematoporphyrinester; (c) chlorine.

photosensitizer reacts with the oxygen to form chemically aggressive, reactive singlet oxygen, which forms organoperoxides by double bonding, e.g. with lipid molecules. These in turn cause the decomposition of the cell membranes by radical chain reactions (Moan *et al.*, 1980).

These two relaxation possibilities are decisive for therapeutic purposes. A further relaxation path results in a non-phototoxic deactivation of the photosensitizer, in so-called photobleaching (Potter *et al.*, 1987). A phototoxic reaction can only result if the concentration of the sensitizing agent is greater than a threshold level. Furthermore, it is important that the sensitizing agent is photostable in order to be able to survive a large number of excitation cycles.

The photosensitizing agent must be excited as effectively as possible, i.e. a loss of the initiating light due to its absorption by hemoglobin and melanin at a wavelength <600 nm must be avoided. Water molecules in turn absorb the photosensitizing molecules in a range >1000 nm. Thus the photosensitizing agent utilized must have its maximum absorption coefficient within the so-called absorption window of human tissue, i.e. between 600 and 1000 nm. The higher the wavelength within this window, the greater the penetration depth of the light into the tissue, up to 8 mm (Wan *et al.*, 1981; Wilson *et al.*, 1985).

Currently numerous photosensitizing agents are utilized, hematoporphyrin, phthalocyanine, benzoporphyrins and chlorine being the most important. To date, clinical studies have made use of the hematoporphyrin derivative photofrin II (McCaughan *et al.*, 1985; Khan, 1993).

BIOLOGICAL MECHANISMS

The exact biological cytotoxic mechanism which takes place during PDT has not yet been fully elucidated. Due to the rapid reaction of the singlet oxygen with cell components and its short lifespan, the cytotoxic process is restricted to the site of the development of the singlet oxygen (Moan and Kessel, 1990). It is diffused over 0.1–0.2 mm under physiological conditions (Lindig, 1981). The differing diffusion of the photosensitizing molecule within the cell leads to a cytotoxic reaction within different cell components. Damage to the plasma membrane as well as to the lysosomal, mitochondrial and nuclear membrane have been described (Moan and Kessel, 1990). Photo-oxidation of cholesterols and phospholipids results in a change in the permeability of the membrane and the inactivation of the membrane-associated enzyme systems and enzyme receptors (Girotti, 1990).

A cytotoxic effect lasting for hours has been demonstrated in *in vitro* studies (Morgan, 1994; Shith, 1994). One may thus assume that the damage to the organelles (e.g. mitochondria and lysosomes) is responsible for this, whereas damage to the cell membranes leads to immediate cytolysis.

In addition to these direct cytotoxic effects, indirect *in vivo* tumor destructive effects and vascular effects could be observed. These constituted an inflammatory reaction on the endothelial cells of the tumor vascularization. The exact mechanism of this indirect cytotoxic reaction is not yet known (Selman *et al.*, 1984).

CLINICAL TESTING

There are only a few reports available on the gynecological utilization of PDT although a large number of patients in various other departments have been treated with it during the past 20 years.

Khan and Dougherthy presented a basic study on the therapeutic possibilities of using PDT for the palliative treatment of cutaneous metastases of breast cancer (Khan, 1993). Thirty-seven women, the majority of them with isolated single metastases on the thoracic wall, were treated. A complete response rate could only be attained in those patients with few metastases with a diameter <1 cm. First experiments were performed with PDT to monitor intraperitoneal metastases, e.g. of ovarian cancer (Sindelar, 1991).

General photosensitization was found to be an undesirable side effect of the clinical utilization of PDT (Pass, 1991). This is caused by the unspecific enrichment of the sensitizing agent within the rest of the body tissue. Initially a specific enrichment of the hematoporphyrin derivatives within the tumor tissue was assumed; this effect on cell lines has, however, not yet been confirmed (Perry *et al.*, 1990). Furthermore, no plausible mechanism for such an absorption is known to date.

This generalized photosensitization is a major limitation for clinical PDT utilization. Hence antibody-mediated PDT – as a possible alternative – has been investigated over the past few years (Oseroff *et al.*, 1986; Rakestraw *et al.*, 1990); the first clinical single case studies have already been undertaken (Schmidt *et al.*, 1992).

ANTIBODY-MEDIATED PDT

A photosensitizing agent with a sufficiently high selectivity for tumor cells that does not cause simultaneous generalized photosensitization is not yet available. Intensive investigations have been underway since the 1980s in an attempt to develop immunoconjugates in which the photosensitizing agent is covalently bonded with a monoclonal antibody. This conjugate has the advantages of only being selective via the antibody and the phototoxicity is only given by the antibody's sensitizer. The procedure is similar to that used in immunoscintigraphy. In our studies we employ two mucine antibodies developed at our institution (Brummendorf *et al.*, 1994).

Hematoporphyrin derivatives are an isomeric mixture and not pure substances, hence these photosensitizers cannot be utilized for the development of immunoconjugates.

There are various types of immunoconjugates for antibody-mediated PDT:

1. direct conjugates;
2. immunoconjugates with a photosensitizer carrier;
3. immunoconjugates with liposome carriers.

Direct conjugates constitute the easiest method of producing covalent bonded immunoconjugates. The molecules of the photosensitizing agent are directly bonded with the antibody via functional groups (Brinkley, 1992). The number of molecules which can bond with the antibody is, however, limited because the antigenic affinity can be reduced by the presence of sensitizers within the antigenic bonding range of the antibody.

The bonding relationship (photosensitizer–antibody) can be increased by using carrier systems with a high number of bonding sites for the photosensitizer. The interventions in the structure of the antibody are thus reduced and the photosensitizer is further away from the antibody, which also helps to reduce interactions (Rodwell *et al.*, 1986; Jiang *et al.*, 1990). Polyvinyl alcohols, polyamino acids and polysugar (dextran) are examples of such carrier systems. Spherical carrier molecules such as polymeric beads and dendrimers can also be used (Bachor, 1991).

Liposomes constitute a particular carrier system. The photosensitizer molecules are enclosed in the liposome which is bonded with the monoclonal antibody. This method not only has the advantage of a high bonding rate, but also offers the possibility of transporting extremely water-insoluble substances without any further modification thereof. The disadvantage of this method is, however, that the conjugates are difficult to get chemically clean and to typify. Furthermore, undesired enrichment and a loss of the photosensitizer as a result of 'bleeding' can also result (Morgan, 1994).

The immunoconjugates developed not only have to meet the prerequisites of the photosensitizing agents; further conditions must also be fulfilled. The photosensitizers must be *in vivo* water soluble for administration and transpor-

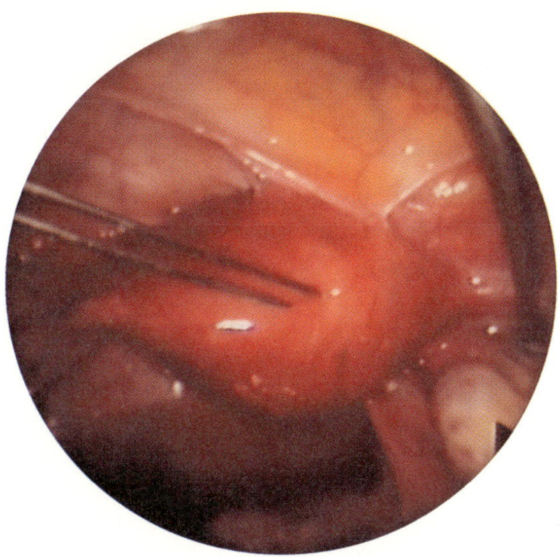

Plate 1 Bipolar myolysis probe in use.

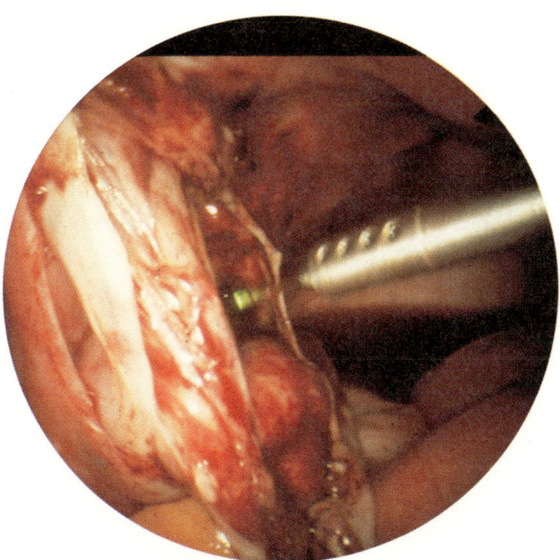

Plate 2 Laparoscopic view of KTP laser photocoagulation of the inside of a chocolate cyst.

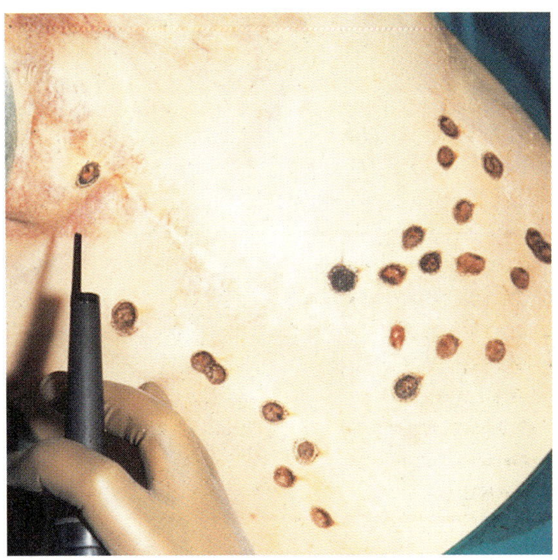

Plate 3 Vaporization of ulcerated cutaneous metastases of primary breast cancer with CO$_2$ laser.

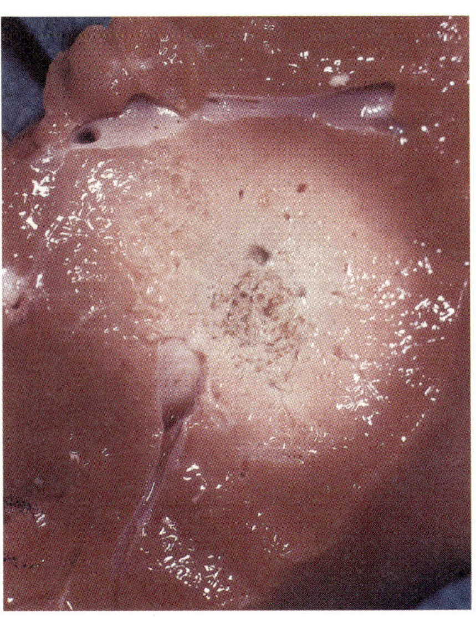

Plate 4 Ellipsoidal coagulation necrosis in pig liver (Ø2.7 × 3.2 cm) after performing an *in vivo* LITT with a Nd-YAG laser and a LITT applicator (3 W, 730 s).

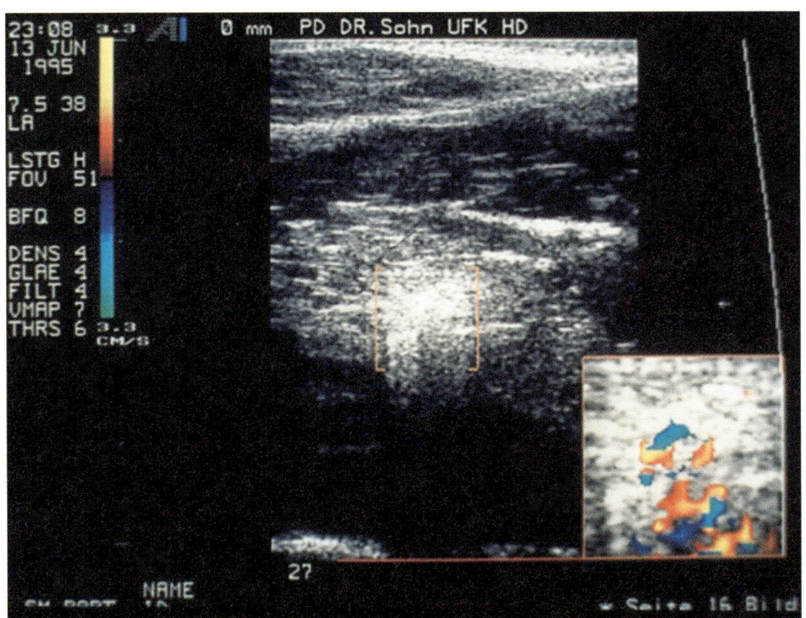

Plate 5 On-line monitoring of a LITT *in vivo* in pig liver. The coagulation necrosis is clearly visible as a hyperechogenic zone.

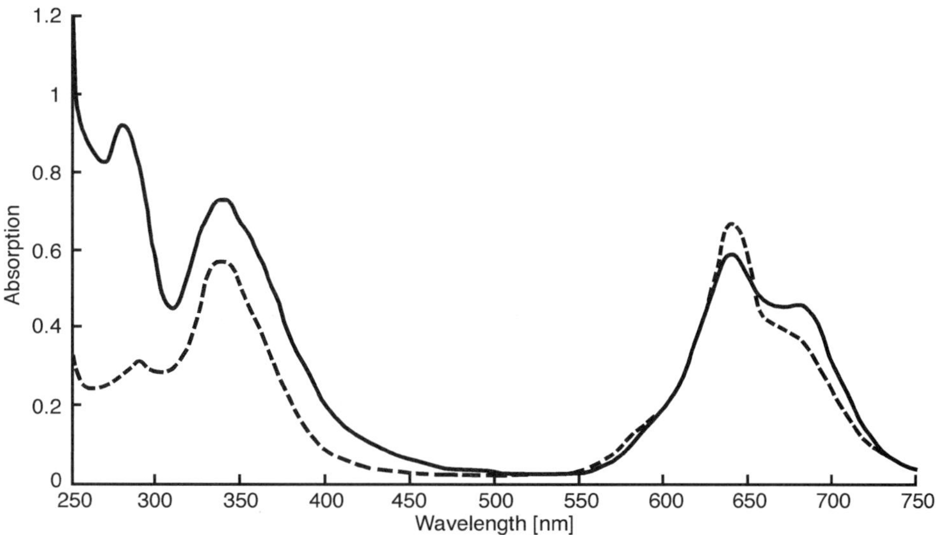

Figure 10.6   Absorption characteristics of conjugated (---) and unconjugated (—) phthalocyanine.

tation purposes (Boyle, 1993; Goff, 1994) and they must have excitable functional groups to bond with the antibody. Furthermore, the sensitizing agent may not tend towards aggregation. Sensitizing agents such as phthalocyanines must be chemically modified to meet these requirements (Figure 10.6).

As far as the cytotoxic effect is concerned, it must be borne in mind that immunoconjugates do not only act primarily on the receptor molecules of the cell membranes, but that they are also absorbed by the cell (Morgan, 1994; Shith, 1994).

In vitro and *in vivo* tests have shown immunoconjugates to have a more efficient phototoxicity and a higher tumor selectivity. The problems as far as clinical utilization is concerned are not only the required chemical modification of the photosensitizer, but also from a physiological point of view the aggregation, the immunogenic effect of carriers and the murine antibodies. A possible solution is the utilization of antibody fragments or humanized antibodies. One must also bear in mind that tumor vessels have a higher interstitial pressure, implying that the penetration depth of the conjugates is limited.

CONCLUSION

The results of clinical case studies with photodynamic therapy carried out to date show that it is possible to utilize this method successfully for the treatment of small nodular metastases (Khan, 1993). The major disadvantage of PDT is the general photosensitization of the patient as a result of unspecific enrichment of the sensitizing agent within the tissue (Pass, 1991). A promising starting point to the solution of this problem is the use of immunoconjugates, in which the photosensitizing molecule is bonded to monoclonal antibodies increasing the selectivity. Experiments have shown an improved tumor enrichment and phototoxicity. The use of carrier molecules to increase the bonding is of great significance. One of the most important prerequisites for the clinical utilization of immunoconjugates for PDT is the chemical modification of the sensitizing agent to enhance the bonding and reduce the aggregation tendency (Perry *et al.*, 1990; Pass, 1991). The immunogenicity of the antibodies can be reduced by using antibody fragments or humanized antibodies.

SYNOPSIS

The three laser techniques utilized for tumor destruction are currently still at different stages within the test phase.

Two techniques – CO_2 laser vaporization and LITT – make use of thermal tissue reciprocal action to destroy malignant tissue. PDT needs laser light for the photochemical activation of photosensitizers.

Only CO_2 laser vaporization is clinically established. Its utilization is effective for the removal of isolated, small, superficial metastases and for supplementary cytoreduction of tumor tissue during abdominal intervention in order to increase the efficacy of neoadjuvant chemotherapy.

LITT is still in the early phase of clinical testing. It appears to be suitable for the destruction of bulky tumors, thus compensating for the shortcomings of CO_2 laser vaporization. The most important prerequisite for the extensive clinical utilization of this technique is the development of effective therapy monitoring systems (open MRI) and the possibility of preoperative planning by means of three-dimensional computer simulation.

Photodynamic treatment is the technique which is furthest from routine utilization. The results of clinical tests to date have shown it to be effective only in the minutest of tumors. Extensive clinical utilization cannot be expected for the foreseeable future, as there are still too many problems with staining, linkage and targeting which must be overcome first.

If one considers tumor biology, where the most important problem is the development of metastases and local recurrences, one may summarize that all three laser procedures will play a role only in palliative treatment of malignancies.

REFERENCES

Anzai, Y., Lufkin, R.B., Hirschowitz, S. *et al.* (1992) MR-imaging – histopathologic correlation of thermal injuries induced with interstitial Nd:YAG laser irradiation in the chronic model. *JMRI*, **2**, 671–8.

Bachor, R. (1991) Photosensitized destruction of human bladder carcinoma cells treated with chlorin e6 conjugated microspheres. *Proc Natl Acad Sci USA*, **88**, 1580–4.

Beuthan, J. (1992) Die laserinduzierte Thermotherapie (LITT) – Biophysikalische Aspekte ihrer Anwendung. *Minimal Invasive Medizin – Med Tech*, **3**, 102–6.

Bhatta, N., Isaacson, K., Flotte, T. *et al.* (1993) Injury and adhesion formation following ovarian wedge resection with different thermal surgical modalities. *Lasers Surg Med*, **13**, 344–52.

Borrelli, M.J., Thomson, L.L., Cain, C.A. *et al.* (1990) Time–temperature analysis of cell killing of BHK cells heated at temperatures in the range of 43.5–57C. *Int J Radiat Oncol Biol Phys*, **19**, 389–99.

Bottomley, P., Hoodless, R.A. and Snart, N.A. (1984) A review of normal tissue hydrogen NMR relaxation times and relaxation mechanismus from 1–100 Mhz: dependence of tissue type, NMR frequency, temperature, species, excision, and age. *Med Phys*, **11**, 425–48.

Boyle, R.W. (1993) Biological activities of phthalocyanines-XVI. Tetrahydroxy- and tetra-alkylhdroxy zinc phthalocyanines. Effect of alkyl chain length on *in vitro* and *in vivo* photodynamic activities. *Br J Cancer*, **67**, 1177–81.

Brinkley, M. (1992) A brief survey of methods for preparing protein conjugates with dyes: haptens and cross-linking reagents. *Bioconjugate Chem*, **3**, 2–13.

Brummendorf, T.H., Kaul, S., Schuhmacher, M. *et al.* (1994) Immunoscintigraphy of human mammary carcinoma xenografts using monoclonal antibodies 12H12 and BM-2 labeled with 99mTc and radioiodine. *Cancer Res*, **54**, 4162–8.

Castro, D.J., Saxton, R.E., Layfield, L.J. *et al.* (1990) Interstitial laser phototherapy assisted by magnetic resonance imaging: a new technique for monitoring laser–tissue interaction. *Laryngoscope*, **12**, 100.

Corson, S.L., Woodland, M., Frishman, G. *et al.* (1989) Treatment of endometriosis in an infertile population: the role of complicating infertility factors. *Fertil Steril*, **34**, 284–8.

Daniell, J.F. and Miller, W. (1989) Polycystic ovaries treated by laparoscopic laser vaporization. *Fertil Steril*, **51**, 232–6.

Davis, M., Dowden, J., Steger, A. *et al.* (1989) A mathematical model for interstitial laser treatment of tumours using four fibres. *Lasers Med Sci*, **4**, 41.

Delannoy, J., Chen, C.N., Turner, R. *et al.* (1991) Noninvasive temperature imaging using diffusion MRI. *Magn Reson Med*, **19**, 333–9.

Deppe, G., Malviya, V.K. and Malone, J.M. (1988) Debulking surgery for ovarian cancer with the cavitron ultrasonic surgical aspirator (CUSA) – a preliminary report. *Gynecol Oncol*, **31**, 223–6.

Dewey, W.C. (1989) Failla Memorial Lecture: the search for critical cellular targets damaged by heat. *Radiat Res*, **120**, 121–34.

Eisenkop, S.M., Nalick, R.H., Wang, H. *et al.* (1993) Peritoneal implant elimination during cytoreductive surgery for ovarian cancer: impact on survival. *Gynecol Oncol*, **51**, 224–9.

Fannin, J., Hilgers, R.D., Richards, R.K. *et al.* (1994) Carbon dioxide laser vaporization of intestinal metastases of epithelial ovarian cancer. *Int J Gynecol Cancer*, **4**, 324–7.

Fiel, R.J., Datta-Gupta, N., Mark, E.H. *et al.* (1981) Induction of DNA by porphyrin photosensitzers. *Cancer Res*, **41**, 3543–5.

Foote, C.S. (1990) Chemical mechanisms of photodynamic action. *Proc SPIE Inst Adv Optical Technol Photodyn Ther*, **IS 6**, 115–26.

Frank, F. (1992) Biophysical fundamentals for laser application in medicine, in *Lasers in Gynecology: Possibilities and Limitations*, (eds. G. Bastert and D. Wallwiener), Springer, Berlin, pp. 349–61.

Gast, M.J., Tobler, R., Strickler, R.C. *et al.* (1988) Laser vaporization of endometriosis in an infertile population: the role of complicating infertility factors. *Fertil Steril*, **49**, 32–6.

Giebel, G.D. and Jaeger, K. (1991) Die Versorgung des fortgeschrittenen Mammakarzinomas, des Lokalrezidivs und des Strahlenschadens, in *Brustrekonstruktion nach Mammakarzinom*, (eds. K. Jaeger and G.B. Stark), Springer, Berlin, pp. 75–85.

Girotti, A.W. (1990) Photodynamic lipid peroxidation in biological systems. *Photochem Photobiol*, **51**, 497–509.

Goff, B.A. (1994) Photoimmunotherapy and biodistrubtion with an OC 125-chlorine immunoconjugate in an *in vivo* murine ovarian tumour model. *Br J Cancer*, **83**, 474–80.

Hukki, J., Lipasti, J., Castren, M. *et al.* (1989) Lactate dehydrogenase in laser incisions: a comparative analysis of skin wounds made with steel scalpel, electrocautery, superpulse-continuous wave mode carbon dioxide lasers, and contact Nd:YAG laser. *Lasers Surg Med*, **9**, 589–94.

Ishihara, Y., Calderon, A., Watanabe, H. *et al.* (1992) A precise and fast temperature mapping method using water protochemical shift. Proceedings of the SMRM, 11th annual meeting, Berlin, p. 4803.

Jacques, S.L. (1992) Liver photocoagulation with diode laser (805 mm) vs Nd:YAG laser (1064 mm). *Laser-Tissue Interaction III. Proc. SPIE*, **1646**, 1–13.

Jiang, F.N., Jiang, S., Liu, D. *et al.* (1990) Development of technology for linking photosensitizers to a model monoclonal antibody. *J Immunol Meth*, **134**, 139–49.

Khan, A.K. (1993) An evaluation of photodynamic therapy in the management of cutaneous metastases of breast cancer. *Eur J Cancer*, **29A**, 1686–90.

Lagendijk, J.J.W. (1987) Physics and technology of hyperthermia. *NATO ASI Series R. Applied Sciences, No. 127*, Martinus Nijhoff, Dordrecht, pp. 517–52.

Lanzafame, R.J., Naim, J.O., Rogers, D.W. *et al.* (1988) Comparison of continuous-wave, chopwave, and super pulse laser wounds. *Lasers Surg Med*, **8**, 119–24.

Lavy, G., Diamond, M.P. and DeCherney, A.H. (1987) Ectopic pregnancy: its relationship to tubal reconstructive surgery. *Fertil Steril*, **47**, 543–56.

LeBihan, D., Delannoy, J. and Levin, R.L. (1989) Temperature mapping with MR imaging of molecular diffusion: application to hyperthermia. *Radiology*, **171**, 853–7.

Lindig, B.A. (1981) Rate parameter for the quenching of singulet oxygen by water soluble and lipid soluble substrates in aqueous and micellar systems. *Photochem Photobiol*, **33**, 627–34.

Lutz, N., Kuessel, A.C., Hull, W.E. *et al.* (1993) A new H-NMR method for determining temperature in cell culture perfusion systems. *Magn Reson Med*, **29**, 113–18.

Mahn, H.R., Nowak, G., Audring, H. *et al.* (1982) Animal experiment comparison of the therapeutic efficacy of tumor excision with a scalpel or with a CO2-laser in subcutaneously implanted louis-lung-cancer. *Z Exp Chirug*, **15**, 38–47.

Malone, D.E., Wyman, D.R., Moote, D.J. *et al.* (1994) Hepatic interstitial laser photocoagulation. An investigation of the relationship between acute thermal lesions and their sonographic images. *Invest Radiol*, **29**, 915–21.

Masters, A., Steger, A.C., Lees, W.R. *et al.* (1992) Interstitial laser hyperthermia: a new approach for treating liver metastases. *Br J Cancer*, **66**, 518–22.

McCaughan, J.S., Schellhas, H.F., Lomano, J. *et al.* (1985) Photodynamic therapy of gynecological neoplasms after presentation with hematoporphyrin derivative. *Lasers Surg Med*, **5**, 491.

Miller, D. (1993) Optical modelling of light distributions in skin tissue following laser irradiation. *Lasers Surg Med*, **13**, 565–71.

Moan, J.M. (1992) Photochemistry of cancer: experimental research, yearly review. *Photochem Photobiol*, **60**, 931–48.

Moan, J. and Kessel, D. (1990) On the diffusion lengths of singulet oxygen in cells and tissues. *J Photochem Photobiol B Biol*, **6**, 343–4.

Moan, J., Waksvik, H. and Christensen, T. (1980) DNA single strand and sister chromatid exchanges induced by treatment with hematoporphyrin and light or by X-rays in human NHIK 3025 cells. *Cancer Res*, **40**, 2915–18.

Morgan, J. (1994) A comparison of direct and liposomal antibody conjugates of sulfonated aluminium phthalocyanines for selective photoinunotherapy of human bladder carcinoma. *Photochem Photobiol*, **60**, 486–96.

Muschter, R., Hessel, S., Hofstetter, A. *et al.* (1993) Laser induced thermotherapy of benign prostatic hyperplasia. *Urologe [A]*, **32**, 273–81.

Muschter, R., Hofstetter, A. and Hessel, S. (1994) Laser induced thermotherapy of benign prostatic hyperplasia – fundamentals and clinical experiences. *Minimal Invasive Medizin*, **2**, 51–4.

Oleson, J.R., Calderwood, S.K., Coughlin, C.T. *et al.* (1993) Biological and clinical aspects of hyperthermia in cancer therapy. *Am J Clin Oncol*, **11**, 368–80.

Oseroff, A.R., Ohuoha, D., Hasan, T. *et al.* (1986) Antibody targeted photolysis: selective photodestruction of human T-cell leukemia cells using monoclonal antibody-chlorin e6 conjugates. *Proc Natl Acad Sci USA*, **83**, 8744–8.

Parker, D. (1993) Temperature distribution measurements in two-dimensional NMR imaging. *Med Phys*, **10**, 321–5.

Pass, H.I. (1991) Photodynamic therapy for lung cancer. *Chest Surg Clin N Am*, **1**, 135–51.

Peled, I., Shohat, B., Gassner, S. *et al.* (1976) Excision of epithelial tumors: CO2 laser versus conventional methods. *Cancer Lett*, **2**, 41–5.

Perry, R.R., Matthews, W., Mitchell, J.B. *et al.* (1990) Sensitivity of different human lung cancer histologies to photodynamic therapy. *Cancer Res*, **50**, 4272–5.

Pogrel, M.A., McCracken, K.J. and Daniels, T.E. (1990) Histologic evaluation of the width of soft tissue necrosis adjacent to carbon dioxide laser incisions. *Oral Surg Oral Med Oral Path*, **70**, 564–8.

Potter, W.R., Mang, T.S. and Dougherty, T.J. (1987) The theory of photodynamic therapy dosimetry: consequences of photodestruction of sensitizers. *Photochem Photobiol*, **46**, 97–101.

Rakestraw, S.L., Tompkins, R.G. and Yarmush, M.L. (1990) Antibody targeted photolysis: *in vitro* studies with Sn(IV)chlorin e6 covalently bound to monoclonal antibodies using a modified dextran carrier. *Proc Natl Acad Sci USA*, **67**, 4217–21.

Rodwell, J.D., Alvarez, V.L., Lee, C. *et al.* (1986) Site-specific covalent modification of monoclonal antibodies: *in vitro* and *vivo* evaluations. *Proc Natl Acad Sci USA*, **83**, 2632–6.

Roggan, A., Mueller, G., Albrecht, T. *et al.* (1995) Dosimetry and computer-based irradiation planning for laser-induced interstitial thermotherapy (LITT), in *Laser Induced Interstitial Thermotherapy*, (eds. A. Roggan and G. Müller), SPIE-The International Society for Optical Engineering, Washington, pp. 114–56.

Sapareto, S.A., Hopwood, L.E., Dewey, W.C. *et al.* (1978) Effects of hyperthermia on survival and progression of chinese hamster ovary cells. *Cancer Res*, **38**, 393–400.

Sava, G., Giraldi, T., Nisi, C. *et al.* (1982) Prophylactic antimetastatic treatment with aryldimethyltriazenes as adjuvant to surgical tumor removal in mice bearing LCC. *Cancer Treat Rep*, **66**, 115.

Schmidt, S., Schultes, B., Oehr, P. *et al.* (1992) Klinischer Einsatz der photodynamicschen Therapie bei gynäkologischen Tumorpatienten. Antikörpervermittelte photodynamische Lasertherapie als neues onkologisches Behandlungsverfahren. *Zentralblatt Gynäkol*, **114**, 307–11.

Seebas, M., Schlegel, W., Wust, P. *et al.* (1993) Thermal modelling for brain tumors, in *Medical Radiology – Interstitial and Intracavitary Thermoradiotherapy*, (eds. M.H. Seegenschmidt and K. Sauer), Springer, Berlin, pp. 143–6.

Selman, S.H., Kreimer-Birnbaum, M., Klaunig, J.E. *et al.* (1984) Blood flow in transplantable bladder tumors treated with hematoporphyrine derivative and light. *Cancer Res*, **44**, 1924.

Shith, L.B. (1994) Internalisation and intracellular processing of the anti-B-cell lymphoma monoclonal antibody LL2. *J Cancer*, **56**, 538–45.

Sindelar, W.F. (1991) Technique of photodynamic therapy for disseminated intraperitonal malignancies. Phase 1 study. *Arch Surg*, **126**, 318.

Stegner, A.C., Lees, W.R., Shorvon, P. *et al.* (1992) Multiple-fibre low power interstitial laser hyperthermia: studies in the normal liver. *Br J Surg*, **79**, 139–45.

Stepanow, B., Blüml, S., Brix, G. *et al.* (1993) Comparision of Tl measurements by means of turboFLASH techniques perfomed on a conventional whole-body MR imager. SMRM, 12th Scientific Meeting, Abstracts, **2**, 742.

Tracz, R.A., Wyman, D.R., Little, P.B. *et al.* (1993) Comparison of magnetic resonance images and the histopathological findings of lesions induced by interstitial laser photocoagulation in the brain. *Lasers Surg Med*, **13**, 45–54.

Van Gemert, M. and Welch, A.J. (1989) Time constants in thermal laser medicine. *Lasers Surg Med*, **9**, 405–21.

Wallwiener, D., Rimbach, S., Pollmann, D. *et al.* (1990) Laser in gynecological oncology. Part I: Experimental results – relapse and metastatic behavior of the Lewis lung carcinoma subsequent to CO2 laser surgery of the primary tumor. An experimental model to compare the effectiveness of various CO2 laser application techniques. *Eur J Gynaecol Oncol*, **11**, 331–41.

Wallwiener, D., Schmit, H., Rimbach, S. *et al.* (1991) Laser palliation of locoregional recurrences of breast cancer. *Eur J Gynaecol Oncol*, **5**, 351–7.

Wallwiener, D., Kurek, R., Pollmann, D. *et al.* (1994) Therapy of gynecological malignancies by laser induced interstitial thermotherapy. *Lasermedizin*, **10**, 44–51.

Wallwiener, D., Kurek, R., Hahn, U. *et al.* (1995a) Laser-induced interstitial thermotherapy (LITT) versus high frequency induced thermotherapy (HFTT), in *Laser Induced Interstitial Thermotherapy*, (eds. A. Roggan and G. Müller), SPIE-The International Society for Optical Engineering, Washington, pp. 542–8.

Wallwiener, D., Kurek, R., Aydeniz, B. *et al.* (1995b) Study of the on-line monitoring by ultrasonography of the spreading tissue necrosis in heterogenous tissue induced by interstitial thermotherapy, in *Laser Induced Interstitial Thermotherapy*, (eds. A. Roggan and G. Müller), SPIE-The International Society for Optical Engineering, Washington, pp. 366–74.

Walsh, J.T., Flotte, T.J., Anderson, R. *et al.* (1988) Pulsed CO2 laser tissue ablation: effect of tissue type and pulse duration on thermal damage. *Lasers Surg Med*, **8**, 108–18.

Wan, S., Parrish, J.A., Anderson, R.R. *et al.* (1981) Transmittance of nonionizing radiation in human tissues. *Photochem Photobiol*, **A62**, 371–8.

Wharton, J.T., Edwards, C.L. and Rutledge, F.N. (1984) Long term survival after chemotherapy for advanced epithelial ovarian carcinoma. *Am J Obstet Gynecol*, **148**, 997–1005.

Whelan, W.M. and Wyman, D.R. (1995) Investigation of large vessel cooling during interstitial laser heating. *Med Phys*, **22**, 105–15.

Whiting, P. (1989) A mathematical analysis of the results of experiments on rat livers by local laser hyperthermia. *Lasers Med Sci*, **4**, 55.

Wilson, B.C., Jeeves, W.P. and Lowe, D.M. (1985) *In vivo* and post mortem measurements of the attenuation spectra of light in mammalian tissues. *Photochem Photobiol*, **42**, 153–62.

Wyman, D.R., Whelan, W.M. and Wilson, B.C. (1992) Interstitial laser photocoagulation: Nd:YAG 1064 nm optical source compared to point heat source. *Lasers Surg Med*, **12**, 659–64.

J.H. Phipps

It is interesting that any candidate for the membership of the Royal College of Obstertricrians and Gynaecologists will almost certainly be able to recite large volumes of data about laser energy in its various forms (Soderstrom refers to this phenomenon as the *Star Wars mystique of laser*), yet few operating surgeons would be able to answer questions concerning that most ubiquitous surgical energy form, *diathermy*. The purpose of this chapter is to explain basic radiofrequency (RF) physics in terms useful to the surgeon.

The principles of behavior of RF energy are of paramount importance particularly in endoscopic surgery, where it is essential to understand that the biological effects of applying such energy may not be limited to the surgical field. Mythology and misconceptions abound whenever diathermy is discussed. 'Never use monopolar diathermy in the abdomen' (Semm, 1983) is a widely stated dogma with little justification or basis in biophysical fact. 'Laser causes so much less scarring . . .', again widely believed and not actually true (Palmer and McGill, 1992; Bordelon *et al.*, 1993). Professor Soderstrom's 'A Watt is a Watt is a Watt' (Soderstrom, 1992) at the cellular level is apposite, but appreciated by few. I make no apologies to my engineer and physics colleagues for what follows; I am perfectly well aware that some points are simplified or

occasionally, to the strict physical scientist, even inaccurate. What is important is that the reader does not automatically turn the page without reading it because of the appearance of equations and arcana which stimulate dim and unpleasant memories of 'A' level physics. This is a chapter for surgeons.

INTRODUCTION

'Diathermy' is actually a term coined in the early part of the century to refer to a quite different application of RF energy – that of heating the deep tissues of the pelvis for the purpose of treating gonorrhea. For present purposes, however, 'diathermy' refers to the application of RF energy for surgical cutting and/or coagulation of tissues. This application has been used for over 50 years and relies on the properties of the passage of RF current at (typically) a frequency of around 500 kHz through biological tissue. The result of current flow through tissue is heating and the exact method used to induce this heating determines the surgical effect obtained (i.e. warming, coagulation or cutting of tissue). The rationale for using this frequency is that current flowing through tissues much under 100 kHz causes contraction of muscle and cellular depolarization, which produces that phenomenon known as electrocution. At 500 kHz

Gynecological Endoscopic Surgery. Edited by C.J.G. Sutton. Published in 1997 by Chapman & Hall, London. ISBN 0 412 58040 3.

(a commonly used frequency) and above, however, the voltage across the individual cell changes its polarity so quickly that the ionic shifts across the cell membrane which facilitate muscle contraction do not have time to occur, as it were. Electrocution does not, therefore, occur when current frequency is very high (as in modern diathermy). Direct application of diathermy to muscle, however, does cause contraction, as any surgeon is aware. This is not a function of the 500 kHz signal but is due to the production of low frequency harmonics of the output signal from the electrosurgical generator, produced as a result of sparking between the applied instrument and the target tissue. If such harmonics are significantly below 100 kHz, muscle contraction may be provoked.

Diathermy generators produce essentially three basic modes of output: monopolar cutting current, monopolar coagulation current and so-called 'bipolar' current. The differences between and the advantages and disadvantages of each mode are discussed below. The general principles and mode of action of diathermy are best illustrated by a consideration of the monopolar mode first.

The difference between cutting and coagulation output is one of waveform. Diagrammatically represented, cutting current is a relatively low amplitude, continuous sine wave where the x axis represents voltage and the y axis time (Figure 11.1). An interesting aside here is that the peak-to-peak voltage of coagulation diathermy is typically 1–4000 volts; the term 'low voltage loop diathermy' for treating cervical disease is therefore a misnomer.

The biological effect of this type of signal in sufficiently high volume and current density at the point of contact with tissue (of which more later) is a very rapid increase in temperature to the extent that the target tissue vaporizes and the surgeon sees a cutting effect. Coagulation waveforms are more complex and vary from machine to machine, but all have in common an 'on-off-on' waveform,

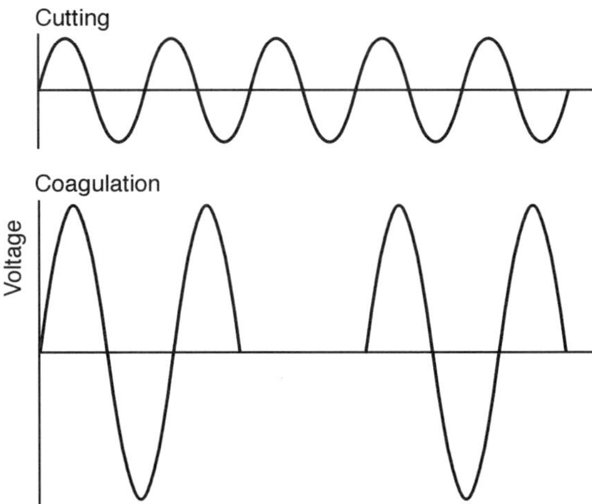

Figure 11.1 Cutting and coagulation waveforms.

where the signal is 'chopped' such that, in cumulative terms, the current is more off than on (Figure 11.1). The amplitude (voltage) of the signal (when in 'on' mode) is higher than that of cutting. The biological effect of this type of waveform, when applied in exactly the same way as the cutting current and at similar powers, i.e. with an identical surface area of contact with tissue, is to rapidly heat tissue momentarily during the 'on' phase, but allowing sufficient time to cool during the 'off' phase, such that tissue does not vaporize and thermal 'spread' is allowed to occur. If the coagulation current is very high, however, this biophysical effect is lost and simple tissue vaporization ('cutting') occurs. The surgeon sees the effect he calls 'coagulation'. The two signals may be mixed to provide an effect which is a combination of the two biological effects (blended current). When coagulation current is applied to tissue such that a small air gap exists between the diathermy instrument and the target tissue, the phenomenon of 'fulguration' occurs. Sparking across the air gap may be used by the surgeon to control ooze from small surface vessels to give a coagulation effect without deep tissue thermal necrosis. This 'non-contact' mode of use of electrocoagulation selectively allows current to flow to leaking small diameter vessels, since the blood within provides a lower impedance route to earth compared to the interstitial tissues. This technique must be used with great care, since without direct physical contact with target tissues, sparking to any vital structures immediately adjacent to the target tissue may occur, although only over very short distances. Moreover, aberrant current flow causing unwanted heating elsewhere is also more likely when the diathermy is activated without direct physical contact with target tissues (see Capacitative coupling, p. 149).

As we shall see later, the signal strength and waveform are not the only factors which determine the final biological effect. Another, usually more important factor, that of surface area of contact between the applicator (usually a surgical instrument) and the tissue, also plays a major part.

TISSUE EFFECTS OF RADIOFREQUENCY ENERGY

Because the voltage which is applied in electrosurgery to tissue is alternating, the current which flows as a result of that voltage being applied is also alternating, at about 500 kHz. To the electrical engineer, the patient may be represented by a resistor and a capacitor, wired together in parallel, which may be referred to as the electrical load (Figure 11.2). Because the body acts as both a resistor and a capacitor, current flowing at diathermy-type frequency (i.e. about 500 kHz) is able to do so through both the resistive and the capacitative components of the body. Although non-alternating electrical current (direct current or DC) is unable to pass through a capacitor, alternating current (AC) is able to pass by rapidly changing the polarity of the charge on either side of the capacitor, which leads to a flow of electrons across the capacitor and therefore current flow. This concept is important, as we shall see. The overall 'ability' of the body or tissues to resist or 'impede' the passage of dia-

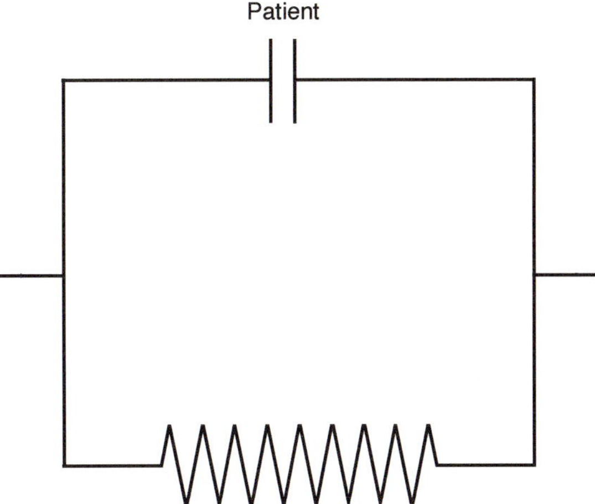

Figure 11.2 Diagrammatic representation of a patient in electrical engineering terms.

thermy current is called impedance. A high tissue impedance means that relatively little current is able to flow through a given structure or volume of tissue (for example, a heat-desiccated pedicle) and a low impedance implies the reverse.

It is an intrinsic property of RF energy at diathermy-type frequencies that the majority of current passes resistively, i.e. only a small proportion of the total current flow passes as a result of the capacitance of the tissue. Does this matter to the surgeon? Unfortunately, yes it does. The concept of current flow (and therefore heating) through tissues without apparent direct 'electrical' contact is one which is difficult to conceive, but which may cause considerable problems (see below).

The surgeon is interested not in current flow but what, in reality, happens at the end of his instrument. The answer is, of course, heating. Although I have tried hard to refrain from putting equations in this chapter for fear of provoking dismissal from readers, I plead necessity for those of Professor Ohm (whose application here, for the serious scientist, is limited since they take no account of capacitative phenomena, but for present purposes serve well):

$$V = IR$$

and

$$P = IV$$

where V is voltage in volts, I is current in amps, R is resistance in ohms and P is power in watts. It only requires elementary algebra to manipulate these two simple equations to explain a great deal about the way diathermy heats tissue. For simplicity's sake, let us equate P in watts (power) as being essentially proportional to 'degree of heating' of target tissues (although in reality the relationship is not so exact or simple). The amount of heating, then, is a product of the voltage applied (V) and the current flowing (I). Let us further assume that the voltage (V) is relatively fixed (this is set by the output of the diathermy machine). It is therefore the case that the amount of heating is directly proportional to the amount of current flowing (I). Going back to the first equation, V = IR, it is easy to see that I = V/R. If V is fixed, then I is inversely proportional to R. In other words, the higher the tissue resistance (remember, we are for the present time ignoring the capacitative qualities of tissue), the lower the current flowing and the lower the degree of heating.

So current flow in tissues causes heating. The biological effects of this are irreversible destruction of cells by denaturation of vital proteins and desiccation. This may be to an extreme and rapid degree, where tissue heating is such that the surgeon sees electrosurgical 'cutting' (i.e. cellular vaporization) or to a slower, more diffuse pattern, 'electrosurgical coagulation'. This sounds obvious and perhaps it is, but the story does not end there.

There is a third type of biologically relevant heating, whose effects are not apparent at the time of surgery but manifest some 48–72 hours later as those of hyperthermia. Mammalian cells are capable of surviving heating to approximately 42°C but at higher temperatures irreversible damage occurs which is both time (of exposure) and temperature dependent.

Irreversible denaturation of cytoskeletal proteins is the first morbid event to occur and begins after about 60 minutes at 43°C. Such 'thermotolerance' time is approximately halved for every degree rise in temperature (Hahn, 1982). Immediate effects of such heating are subtle and cannot be detected by histological examination or enzyme degradation studies if looked for immediately after exposure (Phipps, 1992). Hyperthermic tissue damage is often not taken into account when mapping thermal destruction after tissue exposure to diathermy heating (Duffy *et al.*, 1992), leading to potential overestimation of safety. For example, cases of bowel injury after intrauterine electrosurgery have been reported on a number of occasions (Sullivan *et al.*, 1992) although no overt penetration of the myometrium occurred. Such cases are almost certainly due to hyperthermic tissue damage rather than straightforward burns. Thermal spread beyond the range which is immediately apparent at the time of surgery must always be borne in mind.

RF CURRENT DENSITY, AREA OF SURFACE CONTACT AND FIELD EFFECT

One of the most important concepts to grasp about diathermy is that, despite our previous handling of current flow and heating along simple Ohm's Law principles, we are not dealing with simple resistive current flow when it comes to considering how diathermy behaves clinically. It is at this point that we must draw the line under 'hard' physics and accept that a number of statements about RF energy are true, without exploring the physical and mathematical corroborations which do exist.

RF displays what are known as properties of field effect, typical of electromagnetic phenomena. In practical terms, this boils down to the observation that flow of RF energy does not occur in a simple Ohm's Law fashion, but rather it behaves as a field of energy whose flow pattern is determined to a large extent by the nature of the conductor/conductor interface (i.e. for present purposes, usually the interface between the diathermy-armed surgical instrument and the target tissue in the case of surgical RF use). 'RF loves edges and corners' is an old saying of radio transmitter engineers and understanding this statement is of paramount importance for the surgeon. The surgeon who comes to appreciate this will be better able to use diathermy safely and efficiently. Explanation requires several examples.

The reason why the interface between the diathermy applicator and tissues becomes heated and the interface between the patient and the return electrode plate does not is one of ratio of surface area of contact. The area of contact at the return electrode plate is many thousand times greater than that of the instrument/tissue area of contact, such that the ratio of current density between the two is corre-

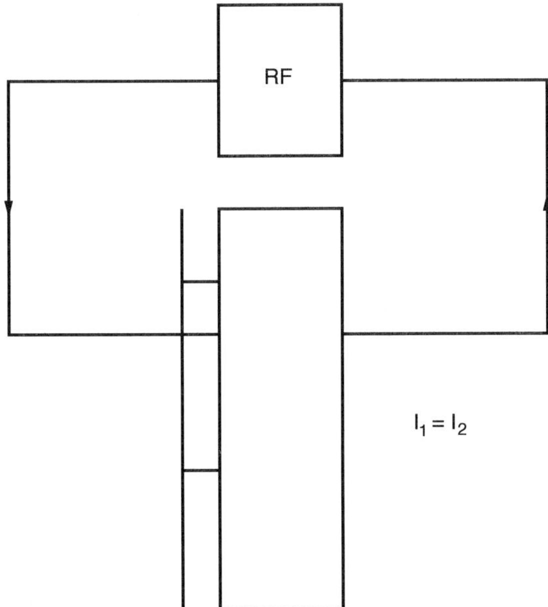

Figure 11.3 Current flow in monopolar diathermy. The area of surface contact is large between the return electrode and the patient, hence current density and therefore heating are very low. The reverse is true for the interface between the active instrument tip and the target tissue.

spondingly high. The same current clearly has to flow between the diathermy instrument and the point of tissue contact as flows between the return plate and the patient's leg (Figure 11.3), but the surface area across which that current has to flow is much smaller in the case of the former. The concept of current density is very important to the surgeon. Anyone who uses diathermy in open surgery will have noticed that the smaller the area of contact of the diathermy forceps with the tissue, the faster and more extreme the heating effect. If diathermy forceps are held in contact with tissue in such a way that the whole of the exposed tip of the forceps is in contact, it becomes very difficult to heat and cauterize the tissue at all. This is a function of current density. Strictly speaking, when RF energy is used to cut or fulgurate as opposed to coagulate tissue, physical contact between the instrument tip and tissue is very brief and disappears once the current is activated. This is because the very small surface area of contact of tissue almost instantly becomes vaporized and the interface between instrument and tissue becomes one of (mainly) steam. Nevertheless, for the practicing surgeon, the concept of area surface contact is a simple and very useful one.

For the endoscopic surgeon, this phenomenon of area of surface contact may be used to good effect when cutting and dissecting tissues using laparoscopic instruments. Many instruments afford the surgeon the ability to create a relatively large surface area of contact with tissue when held in one particular position, such that current density is relatively low when the instrument is activated, but the area of contact is smaller when applied in another position with a correspondingly higher current density. In the former position the instrument effectively coagulates tissue, but in the position of small area of surface contact, the instrument becomes an effective cutting tool. The most obvious example of such an instrument is that flat diathermy hook, but scissors (which may be used to cut or, with the blades closed, as a flat cauterizing surface) are another example. This works to the surgeon's advantage if he is aware of the 'current density phenomenon'. On the other hand, if, for example, the surgeon repeatedly attempts to stem bleeding from a leaking vessel using the very tip of an instrument rather that its flat, wide surface, he will be rewarded with ever-increasing hemorrhage as the high current density of his diathermy application leads to more and more tissue vaporization (a common mistake).

Appreciation of current density phenomena is even more important when one considers 'stray' diathermy. As we have already said, 'RF loves edges and corners'. This means that the potential for high current density on any RF-charged surface will be marked wherever there is an edge or a corner on that charged surface. I am not suggesting that this experiment should be tried but if the surgeon touches an RF-live surface, such as the exposed output pin of the diathermy generator (at low output!) in a bold manner, such that the whole of the surface of his fingers is in contact with the pin, the experimenter will feel very little or nothing. If, on the other hand, he gingerly touches the pin with the very tip of a finger, current will begin to flow via a very small surface area and shock results.

In summary, and in practical terms, the surgeon should bear in mind that a far more significant factor in determining whether a particular diathermy application cuts or coagulates is *area of surface contact*, not whether a 'cut' or 'coag' waveform is applied.

BIPOLAR DIATHERMY

This type of diathermy use has become very popular in recent years and is said to be much safer than monopolar by many surgical authorities, with some justification, although there are qualifications that must be borne in mind when considering bipolar diathermy.

The essential difference between the two modes is that both 'arms' of the circuit are delivered to the surgical instrument (usually

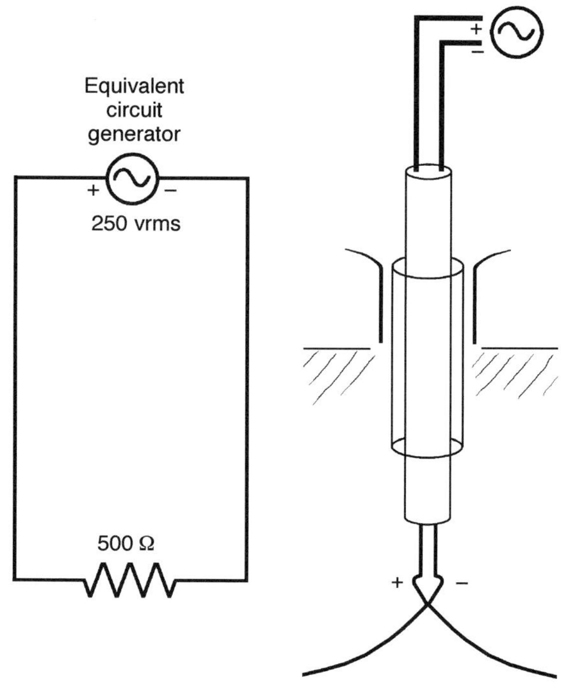

Figure 11.4   Monopolar and bipolar current flow.

grasping forceps) such that no return electrode plate needs to be attached to the patient (Figure 11.4). The great advantage of this is that current flow is largely limited exclusively to the surgical field, since the two jaws of the bipolar instrument are 'live' only with respect to one another. It should be mentioned, however, that under certain circumstances each jaw of the forceps (especially when activated with no tissue interposed between them) may be 'live' with respect to surrounding tissues (Gilbert *et al.*, 1991). It is therefore a point of safety that, in common with all application of any diathermy, *the instrument must NEVER be activated inside the abdomen without good contact with target tissue*. Again, strictly speaking, when fulgurating tissue, or the instant after starting to cut tissue, the instrument and the tissue are actually physically separated by a steam (cutting) or air (fulguration) gap. The term 'good contact with target tissue' is used here to encompass both of these. By 'good contact' I mean that a clear and desirable current pathway from instrument to target tissue is set up by the surgeon. Actual physical contact is not, strictly speaking, an absolute prerequisite, since I am including both cutting and fulguration. This is especially important with monopolar diathermy (see below). The reason for this is that unless the activated diathermy-armed tip of the instrument has a good current pathway to target tissue, a high voltage exists between the instrument and the surrounding non-target tissue (notably bowel), with consequent risk of stray current flow and burns.

The effect of passing current across tissues in such a way is, again, heating. Bipolar diathermy is therefore confined largely to coagulation (although there are instruments which purport to cut using bipolar diathermy, these tend to be of limited efficiency at the present time). Whilst it lacks the flexibility of monopolar diathermy, the bipolar mode is unquestionably safer in certain respects.

It should be borne in mind, however, that tissue heated with bipolar diathermy becomes very hot indeed – around 340°C at the point of maximal current flow – such that a significant thermal gradient is driven by such heating. After 8 seconds of bipolar diathermy application, tissue as distant as 15 mm may be heated to histotoxic levels (Phipps, 1993) due to simple thermal spread when surgically useful power is used.

HAZARDS OF ELECTROSURGERY

The dangers of using RF electrical energy in surgery are the subject of increasing interest and are now commonly cited in medicolegal difficulties which the surgeon may face. It is therefore of paramount importance that anyone involved in using RF electrosurgery (not only surgeons) is knowledgeable about relevant theory and practicalities.

There are any number of ways to categorize hazards associated with diathermy use, but the following seems a logical choice.

CONDUCTIVE THERMAL GRADIENTS

It has already been mentioned that diathermy application leads to heating of a sometimes unsuspected degree and extent. It should be borne in mind that histotoxic spread of heat will always be considerably beyond the tissue boundaries demarked by simple observation of whitening of tissue.

Most hazards associated with diathermy are, however, electrical (Figure 11.5).

DIRECT COUPLING

The most obvious and common surgical error committed with diathermy use is the accidental heating of tissue which is not the intended target ('non-target tissue'). Accidental heating of non-target tissue may occur as a result of two major variable factors. The first is proximity of non-target tissue to the operative site. Clearly, if diathermy is applied to a target structure which lies anatomically very close to

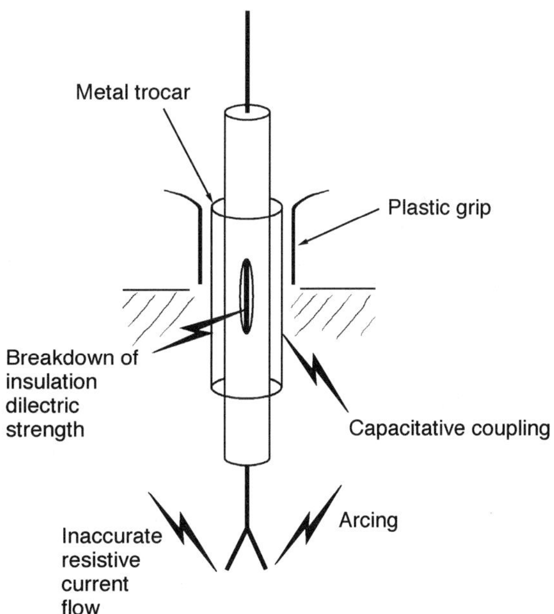

Figure 11.5 Potential causes of unwanted heating and burns, beyond the field of vision of the surgeon, due to stray current flow.

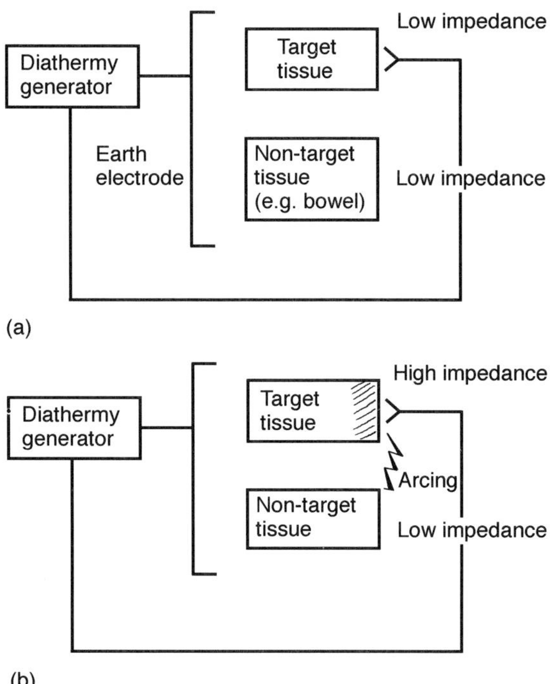

Figure 11.6 (a) Flow of current from the active instrument tip into target tissue at the beginning of current flow, when the target tissue is still fully hydrated and therefore of low impedance. Current flows into target tissue rather than into the immediately adjacent non-target tissue (e.g. a piece of bowel) because the impedance of the two at this stage are identical and the instrument tip is closer to the target tissue than the non-target tissue. (b) Current flow after target tissue heating and desiccation. The impedance of the non-target tissue is now much lower compared to the desiccated target tissue. If the non-target tissue is very close to the instrument tip, current may preferentially flow to non-target tissue and cause burns.

a non-target structure (e.g. a bleeding pedicle lying adjacent to bowel) there is a risk that the non-target structure will be accidentally contacted by the diathermy-armed instrument, resulting in current flow, heating and non-target tissue necrosis (Ata *et al.*, 1993).

However, a second and perhaps less obvious factor, the issue of tissue impedance, once again arises. The example of a bleeding

pedicle adjacent to bowel also serves well to illustrate this effect. When the diathermy instrument is applied to the bleeding pedicle and activated, the tissue impedance of the pedicle and the bowel to which it lies close are roughly equivalent. Current therefore flows exclusively through target tissue and at this stage no problem arises. However, as heating of the pedicle proceeds, it becomes desiccated, its water content falls and its impedance therefore rises. If diathermy is continued, current flow may well occur through the adjacent non-target tissue because the impedance of the non-target tissue, which has not been desiccated, is much lower (Figure 11.6). This is the classic situation where arcing of diathermy current occurs to bowel when pelvic structures such as fallopian tubes are cauterized with monopolar diathermy.

It may therefore be seen, as already mentioned, that it is vitally important that monopolar diathermy never be activated without good contact of the instrument tip with target tissue, with the provisos regarding cutting and fulguration already mentioned. Whenever monopolar diathermy is activated without a desirable earth pathway (i.e. through target tissue), especially during the high voltages seen with coagulation mode, there is always a risk of unwanted current flow and arcing to non-target tissues. There are devices now reaching the market which may help to reduce such risks under certain circumstances, but we shall consider these in more detail under the heading of capacitative coupling.

INSULATION FAILURE

This is a less common problem with the increased quality of insulation used for instrument manufacture and rarely occurs if disposable instruments are used. Clearly, if insulation is damaged or inadequate around the diathermy-charged core of an instrument then there is a risk of current leakage from the instrument to either other instruments (such as cannulae) or, worse, to non-target tissues. The commonest example of this hazard is when the insulation at the terminal end of a laparoscopic instrument is cracked and peels away from the conductive core such that arcing to non-target tissue close to the operative site occurs. It is worth noting that faulty insulation may not be visibly obvious. Even if the insulation is macroscopically intact, it must be borne in mind that one is dealing with relatively high voltages, again especially with coagulation. The ability of any given insulative material to resist current leakage is termed its 'dilectric strength'. When insulation material is repeatedly heated and cooled during sterilization its dilectric strength is invariably degraded to some extent, with consequent risk of unwanted leakage and arcing. The Electroshield system for eliminating these potential risks is discussed later.

CAPACITATIVE COUPLING

This phenomenon has received a great deal of attention recently but the risks of patient injury related to the effect have probably been exaggerated, provided the surgeon is aware that capacitative coupling exists and follows the elementary steps required to prevent any such problems.

Capacitative coupling is a phenomenon which occurs as the result of RF current flowing through one conductor (the conductive core of the diathermy instrument) which is separated from another conductor (the metal sheath of the cannula) by an insulating material (the coating of the diathermy instrument). The result of this is that the system acts as a capacitor, with the insulating coat around the core of the diathermy instrument acting as the dilectric. Charge is therefore induced in the metal cannula body without direct contact with any conductive charged surface. Provided that the metal cannula is in good electrical contact with the abdominal wall, such charge is harmlessly dispersed into the abdominal wall. Because of the large area of con-

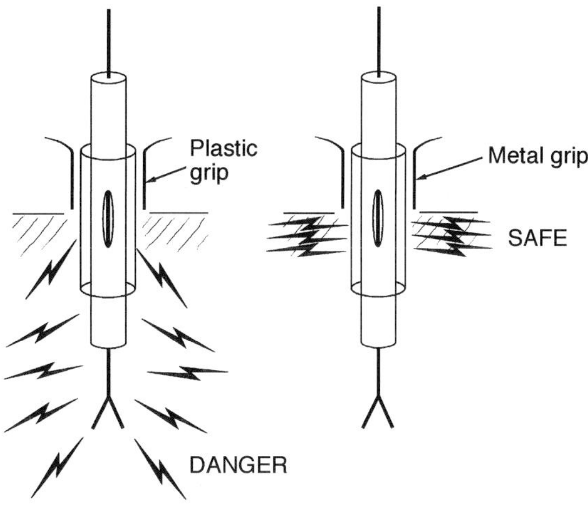

Figure 11.7 Capacitative coupling. The metal cannula may become live every time the instrument passing down its center is activated, because it is sited through the abdominal wall via a plastic (insulative) skin grip. If the area of contact of any bowel touching the cannula is small, as the energy flows to earth current density will be high and a bowel burn results. This problem can be completely eliminated by only using plastic grips with plastic cannulae and metal grips with metal cannulae. Plastic cannulae without special earthing strips must never be used with uninsulated instruments inside the abdomen, such as washer/sucker devices and laparoscopes.

tact of the metal cannula with the abdominal wall tissues, current density is very low and heating is negligible. However, if the metal cannula first passes through a plastic collar in the abdominal wall such that it is insulated from the abdominal wall, any induced charge in the metal cannula body will not be dispersed, since the cannula is electrically 'floating'. It is therefore possible under the latter circumstances that the metal cannula effectively becomes 'live' every time the diathermy instrument which passes through it is activated (Figure 11.7). The worst possible scenario is that during this episode a small area of bowel is touching the metal cannula, which is obviously outside the range of laparoscopic vision. If the area of contact of bowel with cannula is sufficiently small, the charged cannula will earth itself through the bowel with correspondingly high current density and a burn results (Tucker *et al.*, 1992; Voyles and Tucker, 1992). The phenomenon may well be responsible for visceral injuries which may be apparently remote from the operative site.

Two simple measures will reduce the risks associated with capacitative coupling virtually to zero. First, metal cannulae must never be used with plastic collars (gripping devices). If metal cannulae are employed, then conductive metal collars must be used. These allow any charge induced in the metal cannulae to be harmlessly dispersed through the abdominal wall. Alternatively, all-plastic cannulae may be employed, which removes the risk altogether. The second precaution has already been forcefully stated: *never activate the diathermy under 'open circuit' conditions.* Activation of the monopolar diathermy without adequate desirable earthing (i.e. through target tissue) leads to very high voltages between the conductive core of the diathermy instrument and the rest of the patient and also with the cannula body. Such high voltages drive a larger capacitative current flow such that the charge built up in the metal cannula may be substantial and the risks of capacitative coupling resulting in burns are higher.

There is now a device on the market (Electroshield) which forms an isolated conductive sheath around diathermy-armed instruments such that any insulation failure is detected, whether it be direct resistive current leakage (faulty insulation) or capacitative coupling. The instrument shield is connected to a detection apparatus which is linked to the diathermy generator such that any current leakage is sensed and cuts off the diathermy current. There can be little doubt that this device provides the surgeon with the best possible protection against leakage of RF and unwanted heating with consequent burns. Even if this device is used, however, one must never forget that current leakage is only being detected over that portion of the diathermy instrument covered by the detector shield.

Current leakage from the distal end of the instrument, for example, will not be detected unless the whole of the instrument is shielded. Instruments which have a built-in detection shield are now on the market and overcome this problem. It is important to realize, however, that provided metal cannulae are never used with plastic collars, problems arising as a result of capacitative coupling do not occur in practical terms. As far as detection of faulty insulation is concerned, this has rarely been a problem provided good quality and/or disposable instruments are used. The routine use of the shielding technology nevertheless seems desirable.

Finally, one last point concerning diathermy hazards. If activation of the diathermy-armed instrument does not produce the expected effect inside the abdomen within a few seconds, *the generator power must never be increased straight away.* It is essential that all connections are double checked before concluding that diathermy power is inadequate. It is sobering to realize that the most common causes of failure of diathermy are diathermy connection to the wrong instrument (such that the viscera are exposed to diathermy power without visual monitoring) or failure to connect the diathermy at all. The latter may result in horrific injury to the patient. There has been at least one case of corneal burn caused by the exposed pin at the end of the diathermy cable lying on the patient's face with the surgeon standing on the pedal, wondering why his diathermy was not cutting inside the abdomen.

EARTH (RETURN) ELECTRODES

Most modern diathermy machines use earth electrodes which are virtually foolproof, in that a contact-sensor methanism is built in so that the machine becomes non-functional in the event of poor patient contact. Prior to the introduction of this type of alarm system, it was possible for poor patient contact to cause reduced surface area of contact with the return electrode and therefore burns to the patient's leg because of correspondingly high current density. It is obviously good practice always to use a new electrode pad and place it on clean, dry, 'minimally hairy' skin.

PERSONNEL AND EQUIPMENT SAFETY

It is essential that both surgeon and paramedical theater staff have a working knowledge of diathermy. It is beyond the scope of this chapter to describe in any detail safety protocols and theater practice, but a sound working understanding of the physical principles governing the behavior of electrosurgery should underpin both of these. It is important that surgeons bear in mind that, ultimately, they are as responsible for the correct functioning of equipment when applied to the patient as the manufacturer or the service engineer of the equipment. All electrosurgical equipment has to conform to the rigorous standards laid out in the British Standards regulations pertaining to quality of electrical surgical equipment (BS 5724), but faults do occur. Through clever design, most faults 'fail safe', such that machine output is switched off if a problem does arise, although (as we have seen) this is by no means invariably the case. It is the responsibility of the surgeon, where this is reasonably possible, to make certain that the equipment he is using is functioning correctly. For example, it would not be a reasonable defense for the surgeon to claim that the instrument manufacturers or the theater staff were solely responsible for a bowel burn which resulted from damaged instrument insulation. It therefore behoves the surgeon to make certain that he understands (to a reasonable and practicable degree) not only the theory behind his diathermy instrument, but also the practical consequences of that theory.

Hazards to theater staff (including the surgeon) are minimal under normal circumstances, but one or two points should be emphasized. The first is that the diathermy switch (pedal or handswitch) should never be activated until the theater staff have finished connecting the machine properly. Surgical impatience has resulted in more than one ODA's fingers receiving burns. RF burns are exceedingly painful and heal badly because of the penetrating nature of the injury.

A second common practice which should be abandoned is the casual use of metal (non-insulated) instruments to conduct diathermy to the surgical site. Typically, dissecting forceps are used for this to control small skin 'bleeders'. The bleeding tissue is picked up with the forceps and the diathermy instrument is then activated in contact with the dissecting forceps. This should never be done. Most of the time, the surgeon 'gets away with it', because the dissecting forceps are in good electrical contact with the patient and so a good 'desirable' earth pathway is provided (through target tissue). If, however, the surgeon slips and the diathermy (usually high-voltage coagulation current) is applied without good tissue contact, then the voltage may well seek an earth pathway through the surgeon's fingers. If the glove insulating effect breaks down, as it often does (Tucker and Ferguson, 1991), a burn to the surgeon results.

CONCLUSION

In this chapter, I have attempted to steer a middle course between pure physics (which many readers might find impossible to digest) and oversimplification (which invariably leads to inadequate understanding and failure to appreciate how best to achieve safety and efficiency). This has not been easy and doubtless criticisms of my straying too far to one side or the other will follow. However, I hope I have managed to give the workers at the thin end of the wedge, as it were, some sort of intelligible model on which to base their understanding. Readers may find Vancailles' (1994) article on electrosurgery useful further reading.

If I have managed to give at least some readers a working model on which to base their day-to-day practice, then I have succeeded in my aims. I sincerely hope that you have found this useful.

REFERENCES

Ata, A.H., Bellemore, T.J., Meisel, J.A. and Arambulo, S.M. (1993) Distal thermal injury from monopolar electrosurgery. *Surg Lap Endosc*, **3**, 323–7.

Bordelon, B.M., Hobday, K.A. and Hunter, J.G. (1993) Laser Vs. electrosurgery in laparoscopic cholecystectomy: a prospective randomised trial. *Arch Surg*, **128**, 233–6.

Duffy, S., Reid, P.C. and Sharp, F. (1992) *In vivo* studies of uterine electrosurgery. *Br J Obstet Gynaecol*, **99**, 579–82.

Gilbert, T.B., Shaffer, M. and Matthews, M. (1991) Electrical shock by dislodged spark gap in bipolar electrosurgical device. *Anaes Analg*, **73**, 355–7.

Hahn, G.M. (1982) *Hyperthermia and Cancer*, Springer-Verlag, New York, pp. 12–40.

Palmer, S.E. and McGill, L.D. (1992) Thermal injury by *in vitro* incision of equine skin with electrosurgery, radiosurgery, and a carbon dioxide laser. *Vet Surg*, **21**, 348–50.

Phipps, J.H. (1992) Radiofrequency induced thermal endometrial ablation. MD Thesis, University of Leicester.

Phipps, J.H. (1993) Thermometry studies with bipolar diathermy during hysterectomy. *Gynecol Endosc*, **3**, 5–7.

Semm, K. (1983) Physical and biological considerations militating against the use of endoscopically applied high frequency current in the abdomen. *Endoscopy*, **15**, 282–8.

Soderstrom, R.M. (1992) Electricity inside the uterus. *Clin Obstet Gynecol*, **35**, 262–9.

Sullivan, B., Kenney, P. and Seibel, M. (1992) Hysteroscopic resection of fibroid with thermal injury to sigmoid colon. *Obstet Gynecol*, **80**, 546–7.

Tucker, R.D. and Ferguson, S. (1991) Do surgical gloves protect staff during electrosurgical procedure? *Surgery*, **110**, 892–5.

Tucker, R.D., Voyles, C.R. and Silvis, S.E. (1992) Capacitive coupled stray currents during laparoscopic and endoscopic electrosurgical procedures. *BioMed Instru Technol*, **26**, 303–11.

Vancaille, T. (1994) Electrosurgery at laparoscopy: guidelines to avoid complication. *Gynecol Endosc*, **3**, 143–50.

Voyles, C.R. and Tucker, R.D. (1992) Education and engineering solutions for potential problems with laparoscopic monopolar electrosurgery. *Am J Surg*, **146**, 57–62.

INDEX

Page numbers in *italics* refer to illustrations, those in **bold** refer to tables.